CW00631418

Advisory Committee on the Microbiological Safety of Food

Report on

Verocytotoxin-Producing

Escherichia coli

Advises the Government
on the Microbiological Safety of Food

London:HMSO

CONTENTS

EPIDEMIOLOGY OF VTEC INFECTION IN THE USA AND CANADA

EPIDEMIOLOGY OF VTEC INFECTION IN EUROPEAN COUNTRIES OTHER THAN THE UK

CHAPTER 4
VTEC IN FARM ANIMALS

CHAPTER 5
LABORATORY METHODS FOR THE DETECTION OF VTEC IN CLINICAL SAMPLES AND FOOD

CHAPTER 6
VTEC IN FOOD AND PREVENTION AND CONTROL MEASURES

CHAPTER 7
CONCLUSIONS AND RECOMMENDATIONS

GLOSSARY

APPENDIX 1
ADVISORY COMMITTEE ON THE MICROBIOLOGICAL SAFETY OF FOOD
- LIST OF MEMBERS

APPENDIX 2
PATHOGENICITY DETERMINANTS

APPENDIX 3.1
LABORATORY DIAGNOSIS SURVEY

APPENDIX 3.2
AD HOC PAEDIATRIC HUS SURVEY IN THE UK

APPENDIX 3.3
LARGE OUTBREAK IN THE WESTERN USA IN 1992-1993 AND SUBSEQUENT CONTROL MEASURES

APPENDIX 3.4
SURVEY OF SURVEILLANCE/RESEARCH IN SOME MEMBER STATES OF THE EUROPEAN UNION

Spain
  -     Spanish Ministry for Health and Consumption   A.3.4.12

APPENDIX 4.1
METHODS FOR O157 VTEC

APPENDIX 4.2
SUB-TYPING METHODS FOR VTEC

APPENDIX 4.3
SERODIAGNOSIS OF VTEC INFECTIONS

APPENDIX 5
EC AND UK LEGISLATION ON UNPASTEURISED COWS' MILK AND CREAM

REFERENCES

ADVISORY COMMITTEE ON THE MICROBIOLOGICAL SAFETY OF FOOD

WORKING GROUP ON VEROCYTOTOXIN-PRODUCING *ESCHERICHIA COLI*

TERMS OF REFERENCE

The Advisory Committee* decided in 1992 to set up a Working Group and agreed that its remit should cover VTEC in general, as serotypes other than O157 had been isolated from humans and foods. The Working Group began meeting in 1993. The terms of reference of the Working Group were:-

> *"To assess the significance of VTEC as a foodborne pathogen and to advise on any action which could be taken to reduce foodborne disease associated with it."*

*   List of members in Appendix 1

WORKING GROUP ON VEROCYTOTOXIN-PRODUCING *ESCHERICHIA COLI*

MEMBERSHIP

CHAIRMAN

Dr Norman Simmons	Emeritus Consultant in Microbiology to the Guy's and St Thomas' Hospital Trust; Honorary Senior Lecturer in Microbiology, the London Hospital Medical College

MEMBERS

Mrs E J Coleman	Group and Regional Laboratory Manager, Group Scientific and Quality Services, Nestlé UK Ltd
Professor R Feldman	Professor of Clinical Epidemiology, London Hospital Medical College at Queen Mary's Hospital
Dr A M Johnston	Senior Lecturer, Royal Veterinary College
Dr D Old	Reader in Microbiology, University of Dundee Medical School
Dr B Rowe	Director of the Laboratory of Enteric Pathogens, Central Public Health Laboratory, Public Health Laboratory Service
Dr M Stringer	Director of Food Science Division, Campden and Chorleywood Food Research Association
Dame Rachel Waterhouse	Formerly Chairman of Consumers' Association

ASSESSORS

Dr R Cawthorne	Ministry of Agriculture, Fisheries and Food
Mr C Lister	Department of Health
Dr A Wight	Department of Health

SECRETARIAT

Dr V King	Department of Health
Dr R Mitchell	MAFF
Mr G M Robb	Department of Health
Mr T Doole	Department of Health

ACKNOWLEDGEMENTS

The Working Group would like to extend their thanks to the following persons and organisations for their assistance with the Group's work:-

INDIVIDUALS

Dr T J Barrett	Centers for Disease Control and Prevention, Atlanta, USA (Chief, DNA-Based Diagnostics and Subtyping, Foodborne and Diarrhoeal Diseases Branch, Division of Bacterial and Mycotic Diseases)
Dr T Besser	Washington State University, Department of Veterinary Clinical Medicine and Surgery, Pullman, Washington, USA
Dr E de Boer	Food Inspection Service, Zutphen, The Netherlands (Inspectorate for Health Protection)
Dr M Brook	Coppett's Wood Hospital, London
Dr L Beutin	Robert-Koch Institute, Berlin (*E. coli* Reference Laboratory)
Dr M Bülte	Free University of Berlin (Institute for Meat Hygiene)
Dr P Chapman	Sheffield Public Health Laboratory
Professor M P Doyle	University of Georgia, USA (Center for Food Safety and Quality Enhancement Laboratory)
Dr M M Fitzpatrick	University of London (Institute of Child Health)
Dr K Gerigk	WHO Collaborating Centre for Research and Training in Food Hygiene and Zoonoses
Dr P M Griffin	Centers for Disease Control and Prevention, Atlanta, USA (Acting Chief, Foodborne Diseases Section)
Mr B Griffiths	London Borough of Croydon Environmental Health Department
Dr D Hancock	Washington State University, USA (Department of Veterinary Clinical Medicine and Surgery)
Professor G B Haycock	United Medical and Dental Schools of Guy's and St Thomas's (Division of Paediatrics)

Dr M A Karmali	University of Toronto, Canada (Microbiologist-In-Chief, Department of Microbiology, The Hospital for Sick Children and Vice-Chairman of WHO Consultation Group on "Shiga-Like Toxin" Producing *Escherichia coli* with Special Emphasis on Zoonotic Aspects)
Professor R Lacey	Department of Microbiology, University of Leeds
Dr H Lior	National Enteric Reference Centre, Ontario, Canada (Bureau of Microbiology, Laboratory Centre for Disease Control)
Dr A M McNamara	United States Department of Agriculture (Director, Microbiology Division, Food Safety and Inspection Service)
Dr R McNaught	Consultant in Communicable Disease Control, Sheffield Health Authority
Dr J Madden	United States Food and Drug Administration (Director, Division of Microbiology, Centre for Food Safety and Applied Nutrition)
Dr E Mitchell	Department of Health and Social Services (Northern Ireland)
Mr M Mulkerrin	Secretariat, Food Safety Advisory Committee, Republic of Ireland
Dr M A Neill	Brown University School of Medicine and Memorial Hospital of Rhode Island, USA (Infectious Disease Division)
Dr G Reuter	Free University of Berlin (Institute for Meat Hygiene and Technology)
Dr S M Scotland	Laboratory of Enteric Pathogens, Central Public Health Laboratory, Public Health Laboratory Service
Dr H Smith	Laboratory of Enteric Pathogens, Central Public Health Laboratory, Public Health Laboratory Service
Dr J C M Sharp	Scottish Centre for Infection and Environmental Health, Glasgow
Dr P Sockett	Bureau of Communicable Disease Epidemiology, Laboratory Centre for Disease Control, Health Canada, Ottawa, Canada
Dr B A Synge	Scottish Agricultural College Veterinary Investigation Service, Caithness

Dr P Tarr	Children's Hospital Medical Centre, Seattle, USA (Gastroenterology and Infectious Diseases)
Dr R Tauxe	Centers for Disease Control and Prevention, Atlanta, USA (Chief, Enteric Diseases Section)
Dr M Taylor	Birmingham Children's Hospital
Dr E C D Todd	Bureau of Microbiological Hazards, Health and Welfare, Canada
Mr P Van Netten	Food Hygiene Laboratory, Central Public Health Laboratory, Public Health Laboratory Service
Dr S Walker	Campden and Chorleywood Food Research Association
Dr J G Wells	Centers for Disease Control and Prevention, Atlanta, USA (Chief, Epidemic Investigations and Surveillance Laboratory, Foodborne and Diarrhoeal Diseases Branch, Division of Bacterial and Mycotic Diseases)
Dr C Wray	Central Veterinary Laboratory

The Committee also wishes to record its thanks to the Public Health Laboratory Service (PHLS) and the Scottish Centre for Infection and Environmental Health (SCIEH) who provided epidemiological data. The Committee is also grateful to health departments of Member States in the European Union and the many UK Universities who provided information. The Committee contacted a large number of companies and trade associations in the food industry, and other relevant organisations and wishes to record its thanks to those listed below who responded with written or oral information.

Association of Medical Microbiologists
ABP Supplies Ltd
Bird's Eye Wall's Ltd
British Meat Manufacturers Association
Burger King PLC
Campden and Chorleywood Food Research Association
Chilled Food Association
Forte Supplies PLC
Institute of Food Science and Technology
Leatherhead Food Research Association
McKey Food Services Ltd
Marks & Spencer PLC
Milk Marketing Board
National Farmers Union
Perimax Meat Company Ltd
PHLS Working Group on Verocytotoxin-producing *Escherichia coli*
J Sainsbury PLC

Sheffield Health Authority
Specialist Cheesemakers Association
Wendy Restaurants (M & W UK Ltd)
WHO

SUMMARY

1. In this report, we have attempted to assess the significance of Verocytotoxin-producing *E. coli* (VTEC) as a foodborne pathogen by considering published scientific papers, and written and oral evidence from a variety of individuals and organisations. In particular, we have considered information about the sources, routes of transmission, occurrence in animals and food, and clinical and public health aspects of VTEC. We have then attempted to identify the gaps in knowledge about VTEC and action which may be taken to reduce VTEC associated foodborne disease.

2. VTEC infections are associated with a range of illnesses in humans. Verocytotoxin-producing *E.coli* O157:H7 is the predominant cause of human infection, although there is growing evidence that there are many pathogenic VTEC serotypes other than O157:H7. From outbreak investigations, it appears that the infectious dose is low, and illness may occur after the ingestion of less than 100 organisms. Symptoms include diarrhoea, which may become bloody (haemorrhagic colitis (HC)), severe abdominal cramps and vomiting. There is currently no specific treatment for VTEC infection and symptoms usually resolve within two weeks. Public health measures to control VTEC infection are broadly similar to the measures needed to control other gastro-intestinal infections.

3. A small proportion of those with VTEC infection, especially children under 5 years and to a lesser extent the elderly, may develop haemolytic uraemic syndrome (HUS). HUS is probably the most common cause of renal failure in children in the UK and can be fatal or cause associated long-term complications. In a small proportion of cases VTEC infection may also develop into thrombotic thrombocytopaenic purpura (TTP), a condition broadly similar to HUS with neurological complications which affects adults rather than children. From our consideration of clinical aspects of VTEC, we have identified the need for research into factors affecting the outcome of VTEC diarrhoeal illness, the effectiveness of clinical intervention and pathogenicity.

4. Reports of O157 VTEC infections in the UK, based on laboratory isolations, have risen from a handful in the early 1980s to 656 in 1994.* There were peak years in England and Wales in 1992 (470) and in Scotland in 1994 (242). The age distribution indicates that children of less than 4 years have the highest rates of infection followed by the 5-14 and 65+ years age groups. O157 VTEC infections usually peak in the summer months. It is notable that Scotland has much higher reported rates of infection than the rest of the UK, although the reasons for this are not known.

5. Although the UK has a public health surveillance system which is comprehensive by comparison with the rest of Europe and the USA, laboratory investigation of O157 VTEC is not undertaken on all diarrhoeal stool specimens. Approximately half of O157 VTEC infected patients do not have blood in the stools, therefore this is not a logical selection criterion for O157 VTEC examination. Thus, it is not possible to state categorically from laboratory data whether O157 VTEC presents a growing

---

*provisional figure

7

public health problem. Furthermore, there is no national surveillance of HC, HUS and TTP currently being undertaken. We have therefore recommended that clinical laboratories routinely examine all diarrhoeal stools for O157 VTEC and that national prospective surveillance studies of HC, HUS and TTP are carried out. There is also a need to carry out case-control studies during outbreaks to provide better knowledge about sources, routes of transmission, risk factors and socio-economic costs associated with infection.

6.   Farm animals, especially cattle, are considered to be a reservoir of VTEC, but the true incidence and prevalence of O157 VTEC in cattle in the UK are not known. There is also a lack of knowledge about the epidemiology of O157 VTEC infections in farm animals, and husbandry and other factors which may affect herd infection and control. We have therefore recommended that appropriate studies are carried out. We have recognised the importance of hygienic slaughterhouse practices, whilst acknowledging that it is impossible in the short-term to ensure that animal carcases are totally free of O157 VTEC and other micro-organisms. Research into the effectiveness of processing aids such as carcase washes is also recommended.

7.   Laboratory diagnosis of O157 VTEC in clinical, food and environmental samples has developed over recent years with the use of liquid enrichment and the development of methods such as immunomagnetic separation. Methods for detecting non-O157 VTEC remain available only to reference laboratories. There is a need for research into improved isolation media for O157 VTEC, rapid methods to detect VTEC of all serogroups and Verocytotoxin in food and clinical samples. Improved sub-typing methods for VTEC are also needed, especially for O157. We also believe that the currently available methods for testing food and environmental samples should be fully evaluated so that there is consistency of approach.

8.   From outbreak investigations, food appears to be a major vehicle of O157 VTEC infection. A variety of foodstuffs have been implicated: undercooked minced beef products (especially beefburgers), raw cows' milk and cheese, contaminated pasteurised milk and untreated water. Person-to-person spread occurs, probably by the direct faecal-oral route, and this has resulted in outbreaks in hospitals, child care centres, nursing homes, and other institutions. We have endorsed recently formulated public health measures for the control of outbreaks in general, and VTEC in particular, which are essential to prevent and control person-to-person transmission.

9.   We have considered how the foodborne transmission of VTEC can be prevented and controlled. We have recommended that food hygiene measures based on the HACCP system (which identifies those points in the food chain where pathogenic micro-organisms may be controlled or eliminated) should be taken in relation to the storage, handling and correct heat treatment of raw materials, including avoidance of cross-contamination.

10.   We have endorsed the Government's Chief Medical Officer's (CMO) advice, that beefburgers should be cooked until the juices run clear and there are no pink bits inside. We believe this advice should be reiterated to caterers and consumers, as should Government advice on the cooking of minced beef and minced beef products.

Manufacturers and retailers should ensure that cooking instructions for beefburgers will be sufficient to eliminate VTEC. The CMO's advice should be reviewed in the light of the results of the research recommended into the relationship between the colour of cooked, minced meat products, juice colour, the temperature achieved and the survival of VTEC.

11. Manufacturers and retailers should also include labelling information about safe preparation and storage of raw produce which may potentially be contaminated with VTEC. We have recommended that the Government reconsider prohibiting the sale of raw cows' milk in England, Wales and Northern Ireland (the sale of raw cows' milk has been banned in Scotland since 1 August 1983). We have also recommended that the CMO's advice and the current labelling on raw cows' milk are extended to advise vulnerable groups such as children, the elderly and the immunocompromised.

12. Finally, we have recommended that there should be research and surveillance in a number of specific areas. These areas are the acid resistance of VTEC, the effect of sanitisers/disinfectants on its survival, the prevalence of VTEC in raw meats, raw cows' milk and raw milk cheeses, and the relationship between the formulation and colour of cooked minced meat products, the colour of juices, and the survival of VTEC. Knowledge of these areas will enhance our understanding of the organism's ability to cause disease and will allow the development of effective and appropriate preventative measures.

13. The Report's conclusions and recommendations appear at the end of the respective chapters and are drawn together in Chapter 7.

CHAPTER 1

INTRODUCTION

Introduction

1.1 Many strains of the bacterium *Escherichia coli (Esch. coli, E. coli)* are normal inhabitants of the gastro-intestinal tract of man and animals, although some can cause gastro-intestinal disease. Elsewhere in the human body, for example in the genito-urinary tract and in surgical wounds, *E. coli* may also be the cause of infection. Strains which produce toxins harmful to cultured Vero cells (African green monkey kidney cells) are called Verocytotoxin-producing *E. coli*, or VTEC, and these can cause haemorrhagic colitis in humans which usually presents as bloody diarrhoea.

1.2 In 1947, a serotyping classification scheme was developed, based on the identification of bacterial surface structures (somatic/O antigens) which allows *E. coli* to be divided into more than 170 different serogroups.[1] In each serogroup a number of different serotypes can be identified by other bacterial surface structures (flagellar/H antigens). One serotype, *E. coli* O157:H7, is frequently Verocytotoxin-producing. The relationship between *E. coli* O157 and VTEC is represented in Figure 1.

1.3 Throughout this report the following convention has been adopted; when the term VTEC is used, it includes Verocytotoxin-producing *E. coli* of all serogroups; the term *E. coli* O157 is used to refer to *E. coli* of that serogroup, where the precise H antigen type is unknown or not specified; the term *E. coli* O157:H7 is used to refer to bacteria of that specific serotype only, which is frequently VT producing.

1.4 In 1982, *E. coli* O157:H7 was found in patients affected in two outbreaks of bloody diarrhoea in the United States of America, both of which were associated with the consumption of hamburgers. Since that time there have been numerous reports of haemorrhagic colitis associated with *E. coli* O157:H7 infection in North America, Europe and elsewhere.

1.5 It is now known that many *E. coli* serotypes other than *E. coli* O157:H7 are capable of producing Verocytotoxins and causing haemorrhagic colitis. Thus, although to date *E. coli* O157:H7 has been responsible for the largest outbreaks of haemorrhagic colitis, not all VTEC are *E. coli* O157:H7.

1.6 The number of people affected in outbreaks has ranged from less than 10 to more than 700. The biggest recorded outbreak to date occurred in the western United States, principally Washington State, between January and May 1993. It was associated with the consumption of undercooked hamburgers bought from a fast food chain, more than 700 people were affected, and 4 died. The main VTEC reservoir appears to be cattle, but undercooked minced beef is not the only food vehicle.

Figure 1

Schematic representation of relationship
between *E. coli* 0157 and VTEC

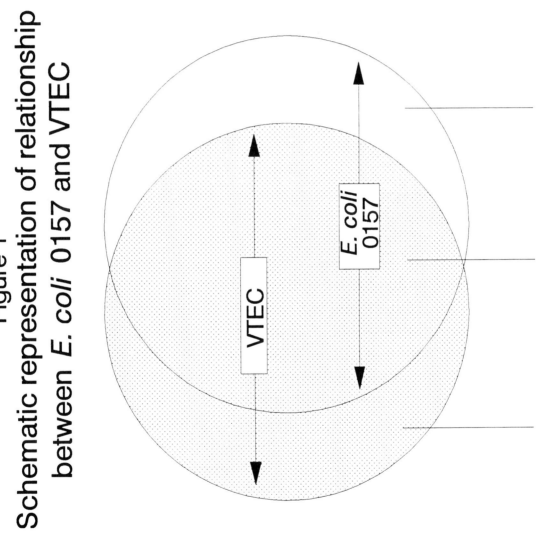

1.7 Outbreaks in the United Kingdom have usually affected less than 10 people and have been associated with the consumption of a variety of foods including minced beef, milk, yoghurt and water. To date, the largest recorded outbreak in the United Kingdom was in Scotland in 1994, when more than 100 people were affected. This outbreak was associated with the consumption of milk probably contaminated post-pasteurisation. VTEC may spread directly from person to person, probably by the direct faecal-oral route, and this has been responsible for outbreaks of infection in hospitals, child care centres, nursing homes and other institutions. Sporadic cases also occur. The number of reported cases of VTEC infection in the UK in 1994 was 656[*].

1.8 A serious complication of haemorrhagic colitis is the haemolytic uraemic syndrome (HUS), a form of kidney failure. Most of those affected are children. In some outbreaks as many as 30% of patients with colitis have developed the disease, but usually the proportion is 2-7%. Nevertheless, HUS is now believed to be the commonest cause of acute renal failure in children in the United Kingdom. It may be fatal in up to 10% of cases and those who recover may have serious long-term impairment of renal function.

1.9 The Working Group on Verocytotoxin-producing *E. coli* was set up by the Advisory Committee on the Microbiological Safety of Food (ACMSF) in 1992, and began meeting in January 1993. Its terms of reference are set out on page 1. The ACMSF agreed that the following key areas of work would be included in the Working Group's review:-

* clinical spectrum of VTEC infections;
* pathogenicity and host susceptibility;
* epidemiology of VTEC infections;
* sources and routes of transmission;
* growth and survival of VTEC;
* effects of food processing on the organism in meat and other products;
* current detection and isolation methods in human, animal, food and environmental samples;
* retail and catering sectors' perspective.

The Working Group has considered each of these subjects in detail.

1.10 The Working Group wrote to food manufacturers, retailers, caterers, trade associations, consumer groups, research organisations and environmental health departments in May 1993 asking for information on VTEC in relation to routine analyses, codes of practice, control measures and research. Similarly, information on research was requested from higher education establishments, and the Working Group considered all Government funded research/surveillance relating to VTEC. A survey of the laboratory diagnosis of *E. coli* O157 in the UK was also carried out. Numerous organisations and individuals were invited to give evidence verbally or in writing and a number took the opportunity to do so.

---

[*] provisional figure

1.11 Following the large outbreak of *E. coli* O157 in the western United States in early 1993, the Working Group sent a delegation to Atlanta USA, to gather information about the investigation and management of the outbreak and subsequent control measures from officials in the US Department of Agriculture, the US Food and Drug Administration, and the Centers for Disease Control and Prevention. The visit was timed to coincide with the 80th Annual Meeting of the International Association of Milk, Food and Environmental Sanitarians in Atlanta where there were a number of presentations on VTEC from US and Canadian experts, some of whom were also involved in managing and controlling the outbreak. Information on VTEC infection in Europe and elsewhere in the world has also been gathered.

1.12 Finally, the Working Group visited a cattle abattoir, a hamburger processing plant, and a range of restaurants serving burgers in the United Kingdom to gain first hand knowledge of the procedures involved.

1.13 The Working Group wishes to express its gratitude to the many individuals and organisations mentioned in the Acknowledgements who have assisted the Group in its work.

CHAPTER 2

CLINICAL SPECTRUM AND DISEASE-CAUSING MECHANISMS

Introduction

2.1   VTEC infections are associated with a range of illnesses in humans. A proportion of infections may be asymptomatic but these may nevertheless represent a source of secondary infections.   The spectrum of clinical disease includes mild diarrhoea, haemorrhagic colitis (HC), haemolytic uraemic syndrome (HUS) and thrombotic thrombocytopaenic purpura (TTP). HC consists of inflammation of the large bowel, with severe bloody diarrhoea. HUS presents as a combination of anaemia, acute renal failure and low platelet count, which may be accompanied by fever. TTP is characterised by fever with skin and central nervous system involvement, and results from aggregation of platelets in various organs.[2, 3]

Clinical symptoms

2.2   The cause of human infection is predominantly VTEC type O157:H7 and most commonly presents as diarrhoea accompanied by severe abdominal cramps, following an incubation period of about 3 days. Vomiting may occur. In approximately half of these cases, bloody diarrhoea (or HC) develops 1-2 days later. Pus cells are rarely found in the stools and fever is an uncommon feature of the diarrhoeal stage of infection. Cases with bloody diarrhoea have a more severe clinical course than cases with non-bloody diarrhoea and may require hospitalisation.[4] Symptoms usually resolve within two weeks. It is possible that there may be a greater proportion of cases with non-bloody diarrhoea than are reported as the illness is milder and patients may not see their doctor or be fully investigated.

2.3   A small proportion of those with VTEC infection, usually between 2% and 7%,[4] but up to 30% in a recent UK report,[5] may go on to develop HUS. Children under 5 years and to a lesser extent the elderly are more likely to progress to HUS. The incidence of HUS in the UK has increased over the last two decades, and is thought to account for at least 70% of acute renal failure in children. The onset of HUS is usually preceded by diarrhoea and although most cases are associated with VTEC infection,[6] other infectious agents such as *Shigella dysenteriae* serotype 1 may be implicated. Up to 10% of cases are not associated with a diarrhoeal phase and the cause is not known. These cases without diarrhoea do not have an identifiable infectious aetiology, have a significantly poorer outcome, and up to 80% may die or develop long-term renal failure.[7]

2.4   Typically, HUS following VTEC infection presents about a week after the onset of diarrhoea. It is characterised by renal failure, anaemia and a low platelet count. Dialysis may be required during the acute phase. Although the progress is generally good in children, some patients may develop long-term sequelae, such as hypertension and end-stage renal failure, in later life.

14

2.5   TTP is best considered as an extension of HUS where in addition to renal failure, the main features are fever and an extremely low platelet count associated with the formation of thrombi giving rise to severe neurological impairment. It may rarely present in the absence of preceding diarrhoea, affecting adults rather than children, and the prognosis is poor.

2.6.   A poorer outcome appears to correlate with a high white cell count in the blood during VTEC related illness.[8] Whilst mortality rates vary in individual outbreaks, the average mortality as a result of VTEC associated HUS infection varies between 5% and 10%, UK [7] and USA [9] data respectively. Although children may die from HUS, a greater number of adults die as a result of VTEC related disease. Deaths occur very occasionally in children and young adults during the diarrhoeal phase, and patients with bloody diarrhoea should therefore be referred to a doctor early.

2.7   Illness does not always follow infection, and there is evidence that those who are of a certain blood group, linked to low or absent expression of a red cell antigen, P1, are more likely to develop severe disease, such as HUS, following infection.[10] Over 70% of the Caucasian population have the P1 antigen and this may exert a protective effect, but further clarification of the role of blood group and of other cellular antigens is required.

Laboratory diagnosis and treatment

2.8   Diagnosis can be made by examining faecal samples for the presence of VTEC during the diarrhoeal phase. Organisms may be excreted in the faeces only for a short period. Serological examination for antibodies to O157 lipopolysaccharide provides additional evidence of recent infection.

2.9   There is no specific treatment. The diarrhoeal phase of the disease is self-limiting and the role of antibiotics in modifying the course of the illness, with respect to duration of diarrhoea and progression to HUS, or excretion of the organism, is not established.[11] Public health measures to control VTEC infection are broadly similar to the measures needed to control other gastrointestinal infections that spread from person-to-person, such as that caused by *Shigella sonnei*. Detailed recommendations have been published by the PHLS in its Interim Guidelines for the Control of Infection with Verocytotoxin-producing *E. coli* (VTEC),[12] and by the Department of Health in its guidance on the Management of Outbreaks of Foodborne Illness.[13]

Infectious dose

2.10   The number of organisms needed to produce infection (the infectious dose) appears to be low, and illness may occur after the ingestion of less than 100 organisms. In a large outbreak due to O157:H7 in the USA in 1993, as few as 40 organisms may have produced disease,[14] and in a recent outbreak in South Wales, only 2 organisms per 25g were isolated from raw beefburger meat tested in the course of the investigation [15] (see Chapter 3). In addition, a report of laboratory-acquired infection from Europe also suggests the infectious dose may be small.[16]

Pathogenicity determinants

2.11   Current knowledge of VTEC organisms suggests that they possess at least two important attributes (pathogenicity determinants) which contribute to these disease processes.

<u>Verocytotoxins</u>

2.12   By definition, VTEC produce powerful toxins, the Verocytotoxins (VTs),[9, 17, 18] so called because they kill a variety of cell types including Vero cells on which their lethal properties were first demonstrated.

2.13   There are two principal kinds of VT:

-        VT1 is virtually identical to the toxin produced by the "Shiga bacillus".[19] In view of this similarity VTs are often referred to as "Shiga-like toxins" or SLTs (especially in North America); and

-        VT2, though similar to VT1 in its biological activity, can be distinguished from it by immunological tests in the laboratory.[20]

2.14   Large amounts of VTs can be detected in the stools of patients with HC and HUS [21] (and also in the stools of patients with non-bloody diarrhoea). VTs damage and, indeed, destroy the intestinal cells in the lower part of the human gut (the colon);[7, 18] as a result, the patient presents with a history of watery diarrhoea. These intestinal cells have lost their ability to absorb the fluid, which is their normal function. When VTs damage the blood vessels of the colon, patients may pass watery stools which have a characteristic bloody appearance (HC).

2.15   Injected into the veins of experimental animals (in which some, but not all, of the symptoms of HC and HUS can be demonstrated), VTs are found to localise in the intestine, the spinal cord and the brain - organs which possess the correct binding sites (receptors) for VT attachment.[22, 23] In patients with severe HUS, damage is localised in the kidney but may also be seen in other organs such as the pancreas and the brain. It has been hypothesised that these systemic effects on distant organs result from blood-borne distribution of VTs to these vital organs. Yet, there is no convincing evidence for the presence of circulating VTs in the blood of patients with VTEC infection or, more importantly, its complications.[24]

2.16   Just as, many years ago, the lethal effect of VTs on tissue-culture cells (such as Vero) was first demonstrated, it is now possible to use other (more developed) tissue-culture lines in the laboratory to demonstrate other VT properties. One such tissue-culture cell-line is HUVEC (human umbilical vein endothelial cells).[25] This kind of cell line is used because it has properties similar to those cells damaged in human disease.

2.17 Recent laboratory experiments with HUVEC cells suggest that when VTs act together with other factors, (e.g. immune mediators which are part of the host's own immune-mechanism), they stimulate VT-target cells (such as those in the kidney) to bind even more VT than they would otherwise do, resulting in increased cell damage.[26] Though these experiments were made on tissue-culture cells, the findings may explain the considerable damage done to the target cells of the kidney in a host animal.

Adhesins

2.18 Experiments in animals have shown that VTEC strains attach to cells of the lower intestine in a characteristic manner, forming attaching and effacing lesions.[27, 28] Several days after attachment, the bacteria penetrate the intercellular spaces with subsequent ulceration and swelling of the affected tissues.[9, 29] Since the normal function of these intestinal cells is to absorb fluid from the gut, their damage results in the accumulation of fluid in the gut contents,[9, 29, 30] and the animals show symptoms of watery diarrhoea. These events resemble the experimental disease of calves infected with bovine strains of VTEC (see paragraph 4.2) and reproduce some aspects of human disease.

2.19 Although these laboratory studies have unravelled some aspects of the mechanism of VTEC adhesion including the contributions made by both bacteria and the host animal, elucidation of all the factors involved in this process of attachment and destruction awaits further studies. More detailed information on pathogenicity determinants can be found in Appendix 2.

Conclusions

2.20 VTEC infection in man may arise from ingestion of a small number of organisms. The most common presentation of symptomatic VTEC infection is diarrhoea, which may be bloody (HC) in approximately 50% of patients. **(C2.1)**

2.21 A small proportion (2-15%) of those with VTEC infection may develop haemolytic uraemic syndrome (HUS); this progression is most likely to occur in children under 5 years and the elderly. Deaths, though rare, are more often seen in adults with VTEC related illness than in other age groups. **(C2.2)**

2.22 The efficacy of antibiotic treatment in modifying the disease is unclear. **(C2.3)**

2.23 Damage to vascular endothelial cells in many tissues by VTs is an important consequence of VTEC infection. **(C2.4)**

2.24 The attachment to intestinal cells by most, but not all, VTEC strains is likely to be mediated by specific adhesins (which have yet to be determined); attachment is followed by tissue damage. **(C2.5)**

Recommendations

2.25 We recommend that all those involved in managing outbreaks make use of the available guidance on the public health measures to control VTEC infection. **(R2.1)**

2.26 We recommend that the Government should consider funding research in the following areas:

- factors affecting the outcome of VTEC diarrhoeal illness, including the role of protective factors (age, sex, blood group) in progression to HUS;

- effectiveness of clinical intervention in treating cases of VTEC infection and HUS; in particular, more needs to be known about the efficacy of antibiotics in affecting carriage, spread of infection and outcome of infection;

- characterisation of the adhesins of VTEC strains, including the minority that do not produce the characteristic (attaching and effacing) lesions;

- *in vitro* methods for demonstration and detection of pathogenicity determinants to aid laboratory diagnosis; and

- the relationship between VTEC diversity in VT and adhesin production and clinical disease. **(R2.2)**

CHAPTER 3

EPIDEMIOLOGY OF VTEC INFECTION IN HUMANS

Introduction

3.1   In the previous chapter on clinical illness and pathogenesis, the range of clinical results of infection with VTEC were described as ranging from none or minimal diarrhoeal illness to acute haemorrhagic colitis (HC), with some individuals showing a post-infectious complication of haemolytic uraemic syndrome (HUS) or thrombotic thrombocytopaenic purpura (TTP).   Although *E. coli* O157:H7 may be a more frequent cause of VTEC illness and infection, there are many VTEC producing *E. coli*, and data concerning the illness associated with them is less complete than that available for *E. coli* O157:H7.   Data about the reservoirs of VTEC are most complete for *E. coli* O157:H7, although there are also limited data concerning some other VTEC.   This background makes it difficult to describe the epidemiological characteristics of all VTEC, and much easier to describe the infection and illness associated with *E. coli* O157:H7.

3.2   The most useful data about the vehicles for VTEC human infection come from outbreak investigations, or from case-control studies of sporadic infections.   In the first instance, the largest number of outbreaks have been associated with *E. coli* O157:H7, and have allowed identification of the vehicles of infection, and study of spread in families, day care centres, and other settings.

3.3   This chapter describes the epidemiological data available in the UK separately from data available in North America and Europe.

EPIDEMIOLOGY OF VTEC INFECTION IN THE UK

Laboratory-based surveillance of *E. coli* O157:H7 and other VTEC

3.4   Although methods used to identify *E. coli* O157:H7 have been modified and their use expanded since the early 1980s, laboratory-based studies of *E. coli* O157 and other VTEC assist in determining whether the problem is of increasing magnitude.   They also provide epidemiological data on age groups at greatest risk of infection and on geographical and seasonal variation in the frequency of infection.

3.5   Studies of *E. coli* O157:H7 have been of increasing scope since 1982, when it was suggested that slow sorbitol fermentation would be of assistance in identification of this serogroup and a method based on this property was introduced in increasing numbers of laboratories.   Table 3.1 indicates the number of laboratory isolates and the rate per 100,000 population from 1982 to 1994 for Scotland, Northern Ireland, England and Wales.   Numbers of isolates have increased from 1 in 1982 in England and Wales to a peak year in 1992 of 470 isolates.   Northern Ireland has only recorded between 1 and 3 isolates per year since 1989.   The number of isolates in Scotland had risen from 3 in 1984 to a peak of 242 in 1994.   The much higher rate of isolations per 100,000 population experienced in Scotland is clearly evident from Figure 3.1.

TABLE 3.1

E. COLI O157 UK LABORATORY REPORTS OF FAECAL ISOLATES AND ISOLATION RATES 1982-1994

	SCOTLAND		NORTHERN IRELAND		ENGLAND AND WALES	
	No.	Rate 100,000 population	No.	Rate 100,000 population	No.	Rate 100,000 population
1982	N/A	N/A	N/A	N/A	1	<0.01
1983	N/A	N/A	N/A	N/A	6	0.01
1984	3	0.06	N/A	N/A	9	0.02
1985	3	0.06	N/A	N/A	50	0.10
1986	4	0.08	N/A	N/A	76	0.15
1987	12	0.24	N/A	N/A	89	0.18
1988	39	0.77	0	0	49	0.10
1989	87	1.70	1	0.06	119	0.23
1990	173	3.39	1	0.06	250	0.49
1991	202	3.96	2	0.12	361	0.71
1992	115	2.25	1	0.06	470	0.92
1993	119	2.32	2	0.12	385	0.75
1994	242	4.73**	3*	0.18**	411*	0.80**

N/A - not available
*   - Provisional
**   - 1994 rates based on 1993 mid-year population estimates

Source: **PHLS(LEP), SCIEH and DHSS(NI)**
Office of Population Censuses and Surveys
General Register Office (Scotland)
General Register Office (Northern Ireland)

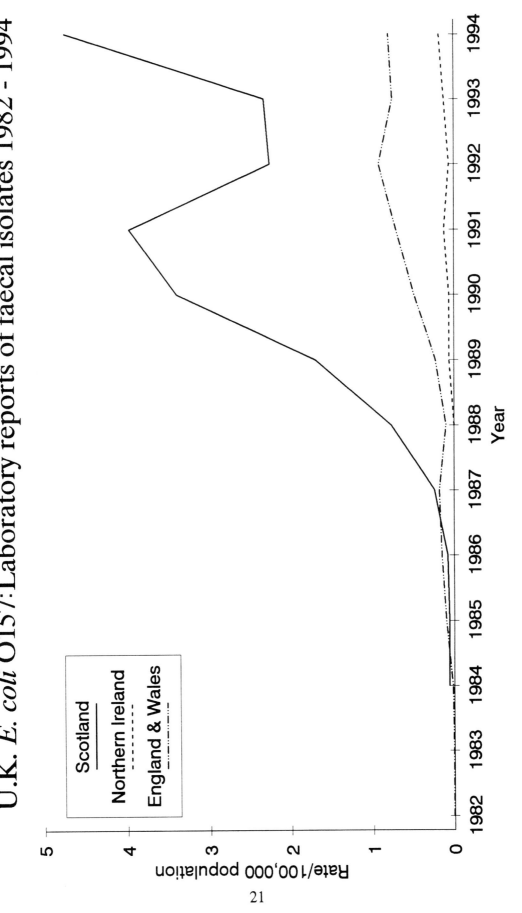

Figure 3.1

U.K. *E. coli* O157:Laboratory reports of faecal isolates 1982 - 1994

Source: PHLS-LEP, SCIEH, DHSS-NI

21

Age, sex, geographical and seasonal distribution

3.6   The age groups of those from whom *E. coli* O157 was isolated in Scotland between 1987 and 1994 are shown in Table 3.2. Comparing rates, per 100,000 population, across the age groups, the 0-4 year olds have the highest rate, followed by the 5-14 age group, and then the 65+ age group. Table 3.3 and Figure 3.2 show the distribution by sex and age group for 1994. Figure 3.3 shows age and sex specific rates per 100,000 population for England and Wales in 1993. The highest rates are seen in the 1-4 age group as in Scotland.

3.7   Seasonal frequency of *E. coli* O157 infections in Scotland between 1987 and 1994 indicates peak months of June and September (Figure 3.4), while the data from England and Wales from 1990 to 1994 indicates peak months of July, August and September, except for 1992 when there was an exceptionally high peak in June (Figure 3.5).

3.8   In terms of geographical distribution, it is notable that some areas of Scotland appeared to have a consistently higher rate of infection than others, particularly Grampian. There is also an east to west split with areas such as Grampian, Tayside, Fife, Lothian and the Borders having consistently higher isolation rates than areas in the west of the country (Table 3.4). Likewise, in England, the Northern, North Western and East Anglian Regional Health Authorities areas have a higher incidence rate (Table 3.5). Wales also has a consistently high rate, but this may relate to an increase in ascertainment as all stool specimens have been screened for *E. coli* O157 since 1990 as part of a special PHLS survey.[31]

TABLE 3.2

AGE-SPECIFIC ISOLATION RATES OF *E. COLI* O157 IN SCOTLAND, 1987-1994

AGE GROUP	CASES	POPULATIONS	MEAN ANNUAL RATES PER 100,000
0 - 4	288	325,105	11.07
5 - 14	150	634,181	2.96
15 - 24	89	753,784	1.48
25 - 34	75	809,061	1.16
35 - 44	72	698,580	1.29
45 - 54	89	580,520	1.92
55 - 64	63	536,887	1.47
65 +	142	768,882	2.30
N/S	13	---	---
Total	981	5,107,000	2.40

N/S = not stated

Source: SCIEH

23

TABLE 3.3

EVIDENCE OF INFECTION IN 1994: ISOLATION RATE ACCORDING TO SEX AND AGE GROUP IN SCOTLAND

AGE	MALE		FEMALE	
	Cases	Rate[*]	Cases	Rate[*]
<1	5	14.77	2	6.23
1-4	31	23.32	40	31.70
4-14	26	8.00	23	7.43
15-24	5	1.30	14	3.79
25-34	6	1.47	14	3.48
35-44	1	0.29	7	2.00
45-54	6	2.11	20	6.76
55-64	9	3.54	7	2.48
65-74	8	4.17	3	1.20
75-84	1	1.09	6	3.58
>84	3	19.06	2	3.78

* Rate = per 100,000 population

Source: SCIEH

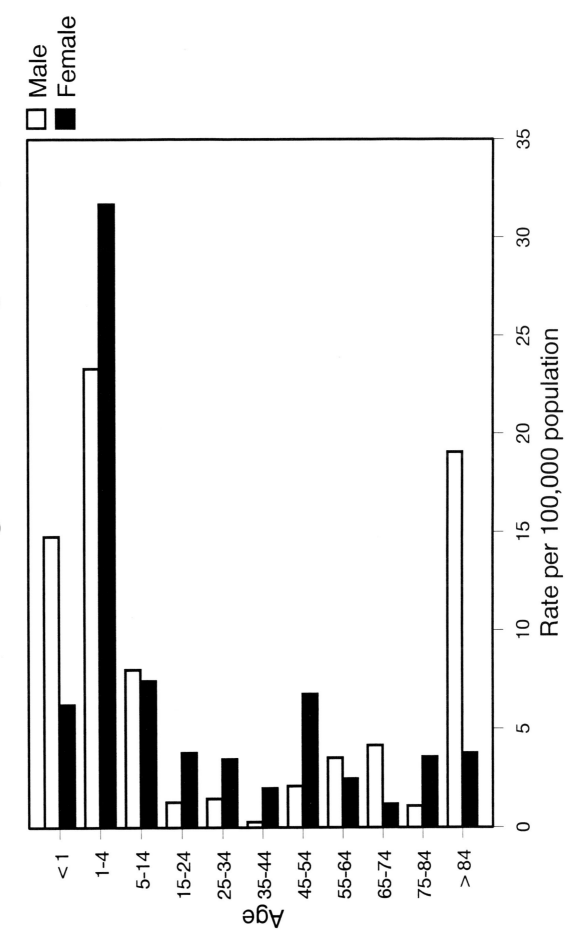

Figure 3.2

Evidence of Infection in 1994 :

Isolation rate According to Sex and Age Group in Scotland

Source: SCIEH

25

Figure 3.3
Evidence of infection in 1993: isolation rate according sex and age group in England and Wales

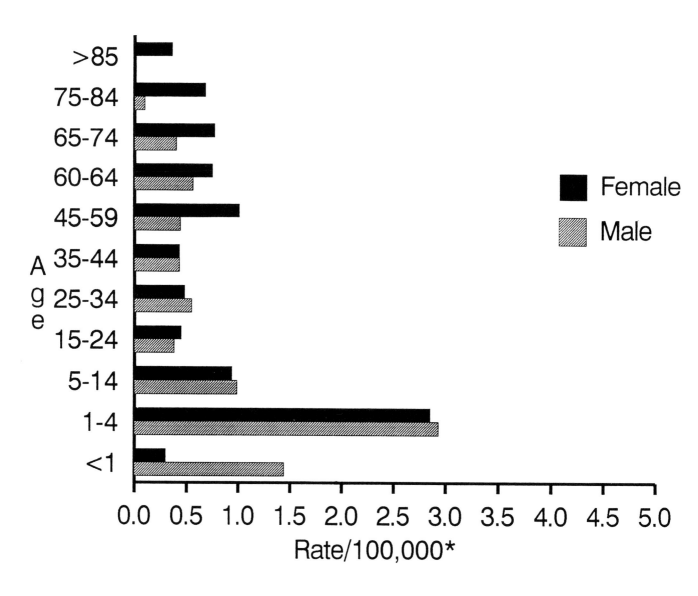

* Figures calculated based on 1989 OPCS data

Source: PHLS

Prepared by: LEP (unpublished data)

Figure 3.4

Seasonal Incidence of *E.coli* O157
- Scotland 1987 - 94

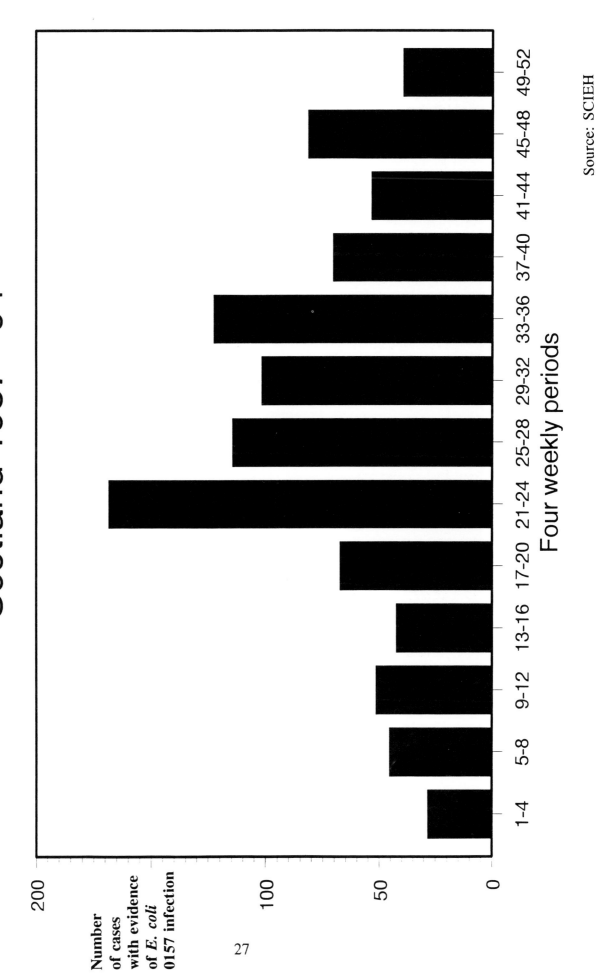

Number
of cases
with evidence
of *E. coli*
O157 infection

Four weekly periods

Source: SCIEH

Figure 3.5

Frequency of VT producing E. coli O157 isolates per month in England and Wales
1990 to 1994

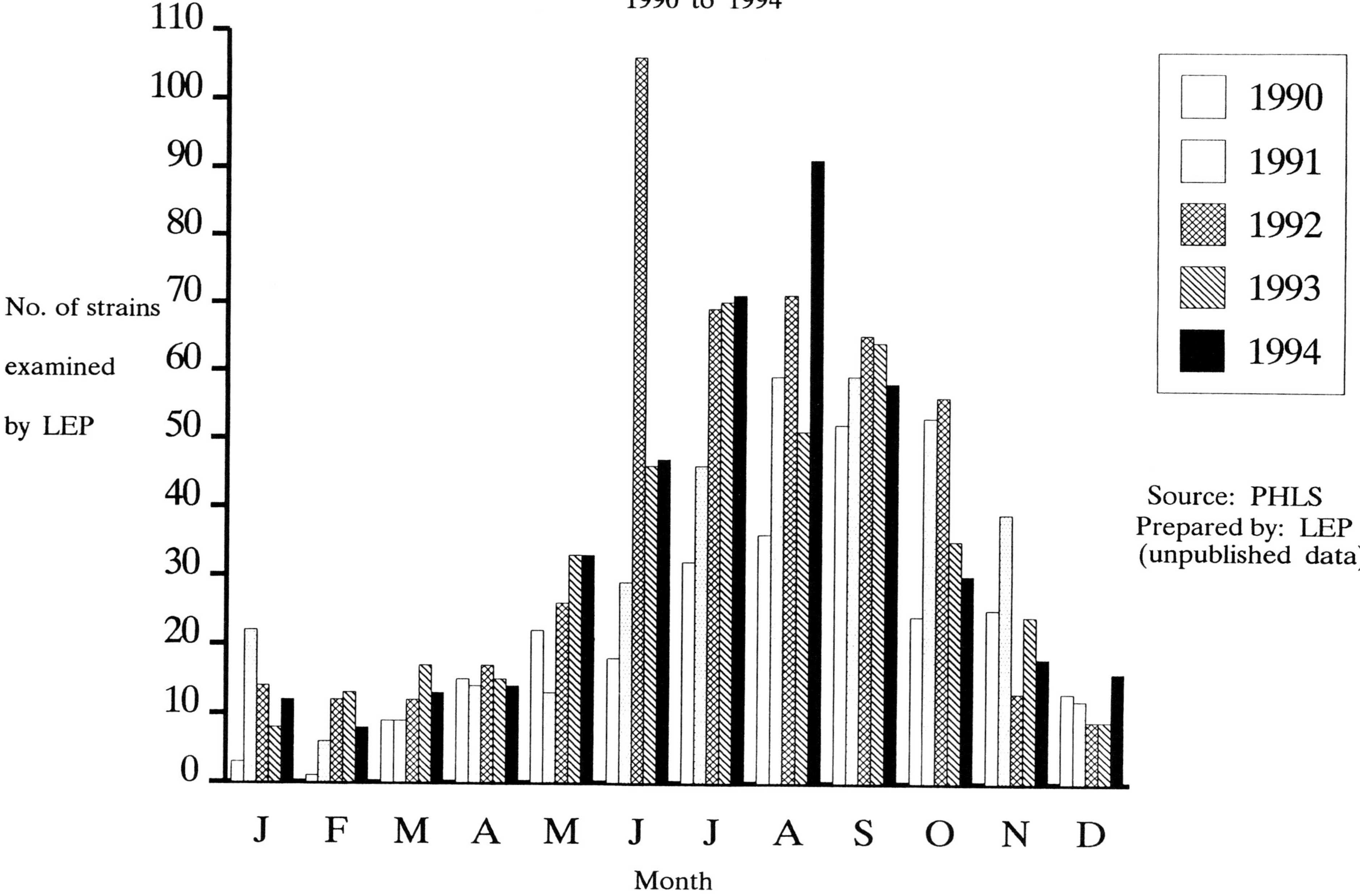

Source: PHLS
Prepared by: LEP
(unpublished data)

TABLE 3.4

E. COLI O157 INFECTIONS AND ISOLATION RATES IN SCOTLAND BY HEALTH BOARD OF REPORTING LABORATORY, 1990-1994

Health Board	1990		1991		1992		1993		1994	
	Cases	Rate *	Cases	Rate *	Cases	Rate *	Cases	Rate *	Cases	Rate *
Argyll & Clyde	6	1.36	7	1.60	1	0.23	7	1.60	5	1.14
Ayrshire & Arran	1	0.27	3	0.79	8	2.12	5	1.33	6	1.59
Borders	3	2.89	23	22.09	10	9.61	1	0.96	0	
Dumfries & Galloway	5	3.37	2	1.35	4	2.71	2	1.35	3	2.03
Fife	15	4.34	13	3.75	9	2.58	9	2.58	20	5.72
Forth Valley	9	3.31	9	3.30	4	1.47	2	0.73	7	2.57
Grampian	46	9.09	67	13.02	38	7.37	42	8.15	61	11.83
Greater Glasgow	14	1.51	8	0.86	9	0.98	11	1.19	21	2.28
Highland	0		0		0		0		9	4.41
Lanarkshire	11	1.96	9	1.60	10	1.78	11	1.96	10	1.78
Lothian	41	5.47	36	4.80	13	1.73	18	2.40	90	12.00
Orkney	1	5.11	1	5.10	0		1	5.11	0	
Shetland	0		0		0		0		0	
Tayside	12	3.05	24	6.12	9	2.29	10	2.54	9	2.29
Western Isles	1	3.26	0		0		0		1	3.40

* Rate = per 100,000 population

Source: SCIEH

29

TABLE 3.5

REGIONAL ISOLATION RATES OF O157 VTEC INFECTIONS IN ENGLAND AND WALES: 1990-1994

Health Region	1990		1991		1992		1993		1994	
	Number	Rate *	Number	Rate *	Number	Rate *	Number	Rate *	Number	Rate *
Northern	33	1.07	25	0.81	47	1.52	31	1.00	54	1.74
Yorkshire	20	0.55	31	0.84	30	0.81	31	0.84	21	0.57
Trent	26	0.55	29	0.61	64	1.35	43	0.91	41	0.86
E Anglian	14	1.04	25	1.20	27	1.29	17	0.81	30	1.44
NW Thames	5	0.14	6	0.17	10	0.29	12	0.34	14	0.40
NE Thames	12	0.32	7	0.18	11	0.29	13	0.34	14	0.37
SE Thames	2	0.05	9	0.24	15	0.40	12	0.32	13	0.35
SW Thames	11	0.37	12	0.40	19	0.64	29	0.97	10	0.33
Wessex	6	0.19	19	0.61	20	0.64	17	0.54	32	1.02
Oxford	15	0.59	13	0.51	50	1.94	21	0.81	25	0.97
S Western	15	0.15	31	0.94	29	0.87	29	0.87	35	1.06
W Midlands	37	0.70	37	0.70	44	0.83	57	1.08	46	0.87
Mersey	4	0.17	11	0.46	8	0.33	10	0.41	14	0.58
N Western	19	0.48	72	1.80	64	1.59	36	0.90	36	0.90
Wales	31	1.08	34	1.18	32	1.10	31	1.06	26	0.90

Data calculated using 1992 OPCS figures

* Rate = per 100,000 population

Source: **PHLS : LEP** (unpublished data)

Laboratory diagnosis survey

3.9   Increasing numbers of *E. coli* O157 isolates in the UK may simply mean that more laboratories are looking for the organism.   In order to investigate this further we carried out a survey of the laboratory diagnosis of *E. coli* O157 in England, Wales, Scotland and Northern Ireland in 1993.

3.10   More than 400 questionnaires were sent to diagnostic/clinical laboratories.   There were 269 replies received, and 252 laboratories reported that they examined for *E. coli* O157.   Detailed results and conclusions of this survey can be found in Appendix 3.1 together with a comparison of the results with an earlier survey conducted in 1989.[32] Information was collected on criteria used for the selection of samples to examine for *E. coli* O157 and methods of microbiological analysis.   Percent positive stools were calculated for different geographical areas using the total number of stools tested and the number positive.

3.11   Approximately the same percentage (95%) of laboratories examined stool samples for *E. coli* O157 in 1992 as in 1989.   Since 1989, some had altered their selection criteria and some had changed to examining all stool specimens for *E. coli* O157.

3.12   The spread of geographical variation in the proportion of stools positive in 1992 was less than that found in 1989: 0.07% to 1.3% in 1992 compared with 0% to 4.6% in 1989.   Ten out of 14 Regional Health Authorities in England, and Scotland reported lower percent positive stools in 1992 compared to 1989.   Oxford still had a high isolation rate (1.2%) compared to other regions but not as high as that reported in 1989 (4.6%).   Those regions that had changed markedly were; Northern with a decrease from 1.2% to 0.3% and Yorkshire with an decrease from 1.5% to 0.13%. The percent positive stools in Scotland had decreased from 1.1% to 0.49%.   Wales and Northern Ireland were not included in the 1989 survey, but both had low percent positive stools for 1992.

3.13   The overall combined percent positive stools for the UK for 1992 (0.4%), was lower than in the 1989 survey (0.7%).   The calculation of percent positive stools for the 1989 survey was based on replies from 130 laboratories and a stool sample denominator of 29,487, giving a mean number of 227 tests per laboratory.   The calculation of the percent positive stools for the 1992 survey was based on replies from 252 laboratories and a stool sample denominator figure of 233,195, giving a mean number of 925 tests per laboratory.   Although in 1992 the percent positive stool samples had gone down compared to 1989, the actual number of isolates of *E. coli* O157 had increased because more stool samples were tested.

3.14   As stool denominator figures are only available through laboratory diagnosis surveys, isolation rates, which are estimations of infection rates, are often calculated using the number of laboratory reports of a particular pathogen per 100,000 population. Calculated in this way the isolation rate per 100,000 population in England and Wales was 0.23 in 1989 and 0.92 in 1992.[33] The results of our laboratory diagnosis survey indicate that it is possible that an increase in ascertainment (i.e. more stools tested for

E. coli O157) caused some of this apparent increase in isolation rate. This conclusion is supported by a total population survey in Wales between 1990 and 1993. Where the mean annual incidence rate and proportion of stools positive showed little change from year to year.[31]

Studies of all VTEC

3.15   Studies of all VTEC are possible using gene probes, although this is primarily a method used by reference laboratories. The advantage of using probes is that a more comprehensive picture is available of the frequency of VTEC in stools. By this means it is possible to identify which serogroups of VTEC are most frequently found in cases of human illness. This information in conjunction with studies of outbreak and sporadic cases allows identification of the most important reservoirs of VTEC for human illness.

3.16   In one survey in the UK during the period 1989-91, VTEC infection was studied using serotyping, Verocytotoxin gene probing and an ELISA for serum antibodies to *E. coli* O157. Evidence of infection was detected in 232, 428 and 615 individuals in 1989, 1990 and 1991 respectively. Of these individuals, 15% were reported as having HUS. Verocytotoxin-producing *E. coli* O157 was the most frequently encountered serogroup, with isolations from a total of 1092 individuals over the 3-year period. Twelve different non-O157 serogroups were identified, the most common being O26 and O145.[5]

Clinical surveillance of HC, HUS, and TTP

3.17   Clinical surveillance studies of HC, HUS and TTP help to measure if VTEC related illness has increased in magnitude in the last two decades. Since these illnesses are serious and often life-threatening, individuals are most often hospitalised, so that hospital admissions data can be used to measure changes over long periods.

3.18   Studies of the complications of VTEC infections are a useful way to study changes over time in the frequency of VTEC infections, but cannot always relate the infections to any particular organism, nor can they focus attention on the vehicle and modes of spread of the organism. Standardised terminology is needed when collecting such clinical information.[34]

3.19   Information gathered about children with the diarrhoeal form of the HUS treated at The Children's Hospital, Birmingham was analysed between 1970 and 1987.[35] The analysis suggested that, over this period, the nature of HUS has changed. From 1982 the rate of referral increased, the prodromal illness more often consisted of bloody diarrhoea, and the mean age at presentation doubled from 2 to 4 years. From July 1983, stool samples were analysed for Verocytotoxin-producing *E. coli* and neutralisable Verocytotoxin. Positive results were obtained in 39% of cases.

3.20 In Aberdeen, 27 paediatric cases of HUS seen at the Royal Aberdeen Children's Hospital from the Grampian region of northeast Scotland between 1978 and 1989 were reviewed.[36] There were 12 cases of HUS admitted between 1978 and 1986 who had a mean age of 3.0 years, while 13 cases admitted during the 2-year period 1987-1988 had a mean age of 7.1 years. The average annual incidence of HUS was 1.25 per 100,000 children 0-16 years old.

3.21 In the British Isles, 289 cases of HUS were reported in a prospective study over a 3 year period.[37] There were 273 (95%) patients who had a prodrome of diarrhoea. It was found that a summer peak in the incidence of haemolytic uraemic syndrome was demonstrated and the 1-2 year age range was most often affected. Evidence for VTEC infection was found in 58 (33%) of 178 diarrhoea associated cases whose stools were analysed, although VTEC were identified in five of eight (62%) patients whose stools were collected within 3 days of the onset of diarrhoea.

3.22 Immunological studies have been used to elucidate the association of VTEC with HUS. In serum from 125 HUS patients, antibodies of the IgA and IgM classes to the lipopolysaccharide of E. coli O157:H7 were found in 55 patients. This improved the detection of infection by this organism by 12%.[38]

3.23 The age distribution of HUS is skewed towards children, which is perhaps because they are most frequently infected, or because they are more likely to become ill if infected. In 1991, a study of the adherence of enterohaemorrhagic E. coli (O157:H7 and other serotypes) isolated from children with diarrhoea, haemorrhagic colitis, or HUS was carried out.[39] Adherence during the first week of life was 13-19% of the adult level - it increased gradually, reaching the adult level at about 4 weeks old. This suggests that perhaps illness rates relate, in some measure, to age of infection.

3.24 It is possible to identify some risk factors for severe complications of infection. The long term (5-21 years) outcome of renal function was studied in 88 infants and children after diarrhoea associated haemolytic uraemic syndrome. After an acute episode of diarrhoea associated HUS, 31% (27/88) of children had an increased albumin excretion, 18% (16/88) had a reduced glomerular filtration rate and 10% (9/88) had both, in association with a higher systolic blood pressure.[40] Out of 72 children with HUS seen between 1969 and 1980 in London, 72% had a history of diarrhoea at onset. Diarrhoea favoured a good outcome among boys but not girls.[41]

Ad hoc paediatric HUS survey

3.25 The British Paediatric Surveillance Unit (BPSU)/Communicable Disease Surveillance Centre (CDSC) surveillance scheme, reported in 1990 annual totals of HUS cases for 1983-1989; these were 54, 57, 83, 105, 130, 104 and 188 respectively. The increase in 1989 occurred in the absence of any change in the method of ascertainment. Clinical surveillance was discontinued in 1990 because of competition for space in the BPSU scheme.[42, 43]

3.26 In order to ascertain if the incidence of HUS has increased in the UK, we wrote to members of the British Association of Paediatric Nephrology (BAPN) requesting data from clinical practice on the number of cases of HUS seen by units over the last decade, and any information on the cause and outcome of these cases. Details of the information collected can be found in Appendix 3.2.

3.27 It was not possible to draw any firm conclusions about the change in the incidence of HUS, particularly in relation to VTEC infection. The information collected was incomplete both nationally and within individual centres and there were no consistent time periods to compare. In most cases no information was provided on cause. Where cause was mentioned some responses referred to *E. coli* O157 and some referred to VTEC. In conclusion, it is difficult to deduce whether the incidence of HUS has changed over the last 5-10 years, but there is a suggestion that there has been an increase over the last 20 years.

Outbreak investigations, and case-control studies of sporadic cases

3.28 Outbreak investigations, and case-control studies of sporadic cases can help to identify vehicles of infection, and allow the study of spread from an index case. In the UK, outbreaks caused by O157 VTEC mainly fall into two categories. In the first category are those involving person-to-person spread, these are for the most part associated with hospitals, nursing homes and other institutions (Table 3.6). A study of an outbreak in 1990 which occurred at a long-stay psychogeriatric hospital in Scotland demonstrated the ability of O157 VTEC to spread from person-to-person, and the need for effective hygiene precautions and infection control procedures in high-risk groups.[44]

3.29 In the second category are those outbreaks which are foodborne. A variety of foods have been implicated in these outbreaks such as raw potatoes (handling), turkey roll sandwiches and yoghurt, but in particular milk and minced beef products.[15, 45, 46, 47, 48] Faecally contaminated water has also been implicated as a vehicle in a number of outbreaks [49] (Table 3.6).

3.30 The largest reported milkborne outbreak of O157 VTEC involving more than 100 people occurred in Scotland in 1994. This was also the largest reported UK outbreak of O157 VTEC. Infection was associated with the consumption of milk probably contaminated post-pasteurisation.[50] Investigation of another outbreak of O157 VTEC in Scotland in 1994 showed that cheese made from raw cows' milk was the vehicle of infection (see paragraph 6.8).

3.31 In using the figures on infection rates, or complications of VTEC infection, it is important to recognize the relative importance of the food reservoir compared to person-to-person spread or spread by other than food vehicles. The dominant mode of transmission in day-care centres is by person-to-person.[4] A study which was reported in 1993 identified person-to-person transmission of *E. coli* O157:H7 as common (median attack rate 22%) when infected pre-school children attended day care centres while symptomatic.[51] Another study showed similar transmission patterns in household members of infected individuals.[52] Although none of these studies measured an infectious dose, they are compatible with a small infectious dose, similar to that found with *Shigella*. Laboratory workers are also at increased risk, as shown in a recent case report.[53]

TABLE 3.6

OUTBREAKS OF VTEC FROM 1987-1994 IN ENGLAND, SCOTLAND AND WALES

Year	Regional health area	Location (reference)	Specimens examined by LEP			Organism isolated	Possible vehicle	Means of identification of possible vehicle
			Number of cases (HUS)	Positive by bacteriology	Positive by serology only			
1987	Birmingham	Community	26 (1)	13	---	O157:H7	Turkey roll sandwiches	e
1988	East Anglia	Community	24 - 1 death	24	---	O157:H7	Handling potatoes	e
1989	Oxford	Community	8 (1)	3	---	O157:H7, PT49, VT2	---	---
	Scotland (Lothian)	Community	4		---	---	Unknown	---
1990	Wales	Psychogeriatric hospital	4	4	---	O157:H-, PT14, VT1 & VT2	---	---
	Yorkshire	Youth custody centre	7	1	---	O157:H7, PT4, VT1 & VT2	---	---
	Oxford	Playgroup	7 (3)	5	2	O157:H7, PT2, VT2	---	---
	Scotland (Grampian)	Community	4	2	---	O157:H7, PT2, VT2	"Water"	e
	Scotland (Glasgow)	Nursing Home	9 (2) - 2 deaths	2	2	O157:H7, PT49, VT2	? Food	e
	Scotland (Lanarkshire)	Psychiatric Hospital	12 - 4 deaths	9	2	O157:H7, PT2, VT2	Person-to-person	---
	Scotland (Lothian)	Restaurant	16 (4)	12	2	O157:H7, PT49, VT2	Food	e
	Scotland (Edinburgh)	Family	5	4	---	O157:H7, PT4, VT2	Person-to-person	---
	Scotland (Edinburgh)	Nursing Home	5	5	---	O157:H7, PT49, VT2	? Food	e

TABLE 3.6 - *Continued*

			Specimens examined by LEP					
Year	Regional health area	Location (reference)	Number of cases (HUS)	Positive by bacteriology	Positive by serology only	Organism isolated	Possible vehicle	Means of identification of possible vehicle
1991	NW England (Scotland, Oxford)	Fast food chains	23 (3)	21	1	O157:H7, PT31, VT2 *	? Food	a
	Oxford	School trip to Austria	6	6	--	O157:H7, PT49, VT2	--	--
	NW England	Community	17 (5)	16	1	O157:H7, PT49, VT2	--	--
	Wales (Carmarthen)	Nursery	10	10	--	O157:H-, PT49, VT2	--	--
	Scotland (Borders)	Eventide homes, community	21	20	1	O157:H7, PT1, VT1 & VT2	? Butcher meat	e
	Scotland (Aberdeen)	Restaurant	6	6	--	O157:H7, PT32, VT2	--	--
	Scotland (Lothian)	Community	5 (2)	5	--	O157:H7, PT2, VT2	Delicatessen	e
1992	NW England	Psychiatric hospital	14 - 3 deaths	4	1	O157:H7, PT2, VT1 & VT2	--	--
	Trent	Nursing Home	5	5	--	O157:H7, PT2, VT2	--	--
	Scotland (Borders)	Playgroup	6	6	--	O157:H7, PT49, VT2	? Paddling pool	e
	Oxford (Northampton)	Nursery	35 (5)	26	2	O157:H7, PT2, VT2	--	--
	Trent	Public House	3 - 1 death	3	--	O157:H7, PT2, VT2	--	--
	Wessex	Scout camp	3	3	--	O157:H7, PT2, VT2	--	--
	Scotland (Glasgow)	Hospital	6	5	1	O157:H7, PT1, VT1 & VT2	Person-to-person	
1993	England (Sheffield)	Community	11 (3)	6	--	O157:H7, PT2, VT2	Raw milk	m
	W Midlands	Factory function	7 (2)	4	--	O157:H7, PT49, VT2	--	--
	Various[1]	Community	4	4	--	O157:H7, PT28, VT2	--	--
	London	Community	5	5	--	O157:H7, PT2, VT2	Raw burger	m
	Yorkshire	Community	9	9	--	O157:H7, PT49, VT2	--	--
	Wales (Gwent)	Community	8 (1)	8	--	O157:H7, PT49, VT2	Beef burgers	m

TABLE 3.6 - *Continued*

Year	Regional health area	Location (reference)	Number of cases (HUS)	Specimens examined by LEP		Organism isolated	Possible vehicle	Means of identification of possible vehicle
				Positive by bacteriology	Positive by serology only			
1994	Wales	Farm	2	1	---	O157:H-, PT4, VT2	---	---
	Various	Visited Majorca	5	5	---	O157:H-, PT-RDNC, VT2	---	---
	Scotland (East Kilbride)	Birthday	7 (3)	2	2	O157:H7, PT2, VT2	Person-to-person	---
	Scotland (Coatbridge)	Community	4 (2)	2	2	O157:H7, PT49, VT2	Unknown	---
	Scotland (Fife)	Community	19 (1)	8		O157:H7, PT4, VT1 & VT2	Butcher meat	e
	Scotland (West Lothian)	Community	>100 (9) - 1 death	69	1	O157:H7, PT2, VT	"Pasteurised" milk	m

a = anecdotal
e = epidemiological
m = microbiological
* = organism isolated was urease positive
RDNC: reacts does not conform
1 = O157 VTEC PT28 isolated in Harrogate, Leeds, Portsmouth and Guildford

Source: **PHLS-LEP**
SCIEH

Compiled by: **DH**

EPIDEMIOLOGY OF VTEC INFECTION IN THE USA AND CANADA

Surveillance: laboratory-based studies

3.32   There is no data on incidence over time of *E. coli* O157 infections in the US as a nationwide laboratory-based surveillance system has only existed since 1 January 1994. The Centers for Disease Control and Prevention (CDC) Atlanta have no records of outbreaks of bloody diarrhoea of unknown origin before 1982 and in a review of over 3,000 *E. coli* strains serotyped between 1973 and 1983 only one was identified as *E. coli* O157.[54] This suggests that *E. coli* O157 was not likely to have been a frequent aetiological agent of bloody diarrhoea in the US before 1982.

3.33   In Canada, many laboratories screen for *E. coli* O157 in bloody and non-bloody diarrhoea.[55] An isolation rate of 5.2/100,000 population was recorded in 1987 which increased to 8.8 in 1989 and then decreased to 5.6 in 1991 (Table 3.7).

3.34   A number of studies both in Canada and the US have compared the isolation rate of *E. coli* O157 with other enteropathogens and found it to be the second or third most frequently isolated organism, and more common than *Shigella*.[56]

3.35   In an extended US study of 52 patients, (predominantly children with post-diarrhoeal HUS), a timeline was produced for each patient. The timeline included onset of symptoms, date of culture which detected *E. coli* O157:H7, and onset of HUS. It was possible to recover the pathogen in 24 (96%) of 25 patients whose stools were appropriately tested during the first six days of illness.[57]

3.36   In order to determine the prevalence of *E. coli* O157 infections, 10 study hospitals throughout the US cultured all stool specimens (26,239) using the same isolation methodology over 2 years. *E. coli* O157 was isolated from 0.4% of specimens compared with *Campylobacter* 2.2%; *Salmonella* 1.8% and *Shigella* 1.0%. *E. coli* O157 was isolated from 7.8% of specimens with visible blood, more than *Campylobacter* (5.7%), *Salmonella* (3.4%), or *Shigella* (3.6%). Only 68% of isolates were from specimens with visible blood.[58] The same study found eating hamburgers (rare or pink), hot dogs and meals at fast food restaurants all to be risk factors for *E. coli* O157 infection.

Age, geographical and seasonal distribution

3.37   In the same US study, *E. coli* O157:H7 was isolated more frequently at hospitals in the northern and western states than in the southern states. Infections appeared to peak in the summer; Washington State recorded a peak between June and August in 1987.[59] The age groups with the highest number of isolates were 0-9 years and > 60 years.[58] However, when stool samples were used as a denominator, then the 50-59 years age group had the highest percentage positive stools (1.0%).

3.38   In Canada, the geographical distribution according to number of isolations of *E. coli* O157 varies from province-to-province (Table 3.8). When this is converted to isolation rate Alberta has the highest, peaking at over 15.0/100,000 population in 1989. The seasonal distribution of infection is similar to that seen in the US and UK, with a peak in July and August (personal communication Dr H Lior). The age range affected is from 3 months to 83 years with isolation rates of 40/100,000 in 0-4 years, 3.5/100,000 in 45-65 years and 14.5/100,000 in those over 65 years.[60]

TABLE 3.7

**VTEC IN CANADA: LABORATORY ISOLATIONS REPORTED TO LCDC
1982-1993, ANNUAL TOTALS AND REPORTING RATES**

YEAR	POPULATION IN MILLIONS	VTEC	RATE PER 100,000
1982	25.20	25	0.10
1983	25.46	59	0.23
1984	25.70	163	0.63
1985	25.94	294	1.13
1986	26.20	750	2.86
1987	26.55	1,381	5.20
1988	26.89	1,785	6.63
1989	27.38	2,407	8.79
1990	27.79	1,585	5.70
1991	28.12	1,565	5.57
1992	28.44	1,642	5.77
1993	28.75	1,166	4.06

Prepared by the Laboratory Centre for Disease Control (LCDC) with acknowledgement to Dr H Lior, Dr J Hockin and Statistics Canada (Population estimates).

TABLE 3.8

VTEC IN CANADA: LABORATORY ISOLATIONS REPORTED TO LCDC
1988-1993, ANNUAL TOTALS BY PROVINCE

PROVINCE	1988	1989	1990	1991	1992	1993
British Columbia	342	403	247	182	296	158
Alberta	296	376	247	198	356	152
Saskatchewan	101	116	48	51	59	50
Manitoba	57	190	52	226	74	90
Ontario	659	796	707	558	434	386
Quebec	199	389	145	248	320	273
New Brunswick	29	60	36	36	43	20
Nova Scotia	43	46	63	36	24	19
Prince Edward Island	10	5	30	26	23	11
Newfoundland	49	26	10	4	13	7

Prepared by the Laboratory Centre for Disease Control (LCDC) with acknowledgement to Dr H Lior, Dr J Hockin and Statistics Canada (Population estimates).

TABLE 3.9

REPORTED OUTBREAKS OF *E. COLI* O157:H7 INFECTION IN THE USA 1982-1993

Month and year	State[+]	Setting	No. affected	No. hospitalised	No. with HUS or TTP*	No. dead	Likely vehicle or mode of spread
February 1982	OR	Community	26	19	0	0	Ground beef
May 1982	MI	Community	21	14	0	0	Ground beef
September 1984	NE	Nursing home	34	14	1	4	Ground beef
September 1984	NC	Day-care centre	36	3	3	0	Person-to-person
October 1986	WA	Community	37	17	4	2	Ground beef/ranch dressing
June 1987	UT	Custodial institutions	51	8	8	4	Ground beef/person-to-person
May 1988	WI	School	61	2	0	0	Roast beef
August 1988	MN	Day-care centre	19	NR	3	0	Person-to-person
October 1988	MN	School	54	4	0	0	Pre-cooked ground beef
December 1989	MO	Community	243	32	2	4	Municipal water
July 1990	ND	Community	65	16	2	0	Roast beef
November 1990	MT	School	10	2	1	0	School Lunch
July 1991	OR	Community	28	7	3	0	Swimming water
November 1991	MA	Community	23	7	3	0	Apple cider
July 1992	NV	Day-care centre	57	1	0	0	Person-to-person
September 1992	ME	Family	4	3	1	1	Vegetable/person-to-person
December 1992	OR	Community	8	2	0	0	Raw milk
January 1993	WA, ID, NV,CA	Community	732	195	55	4	Ground beef
March 1993	OR	Community	48	12	0	0	Mayonnaise-containing dressing and sauces

* HUS = Haemolytic Uraemic Syndrome, TTP = Thrombotic Thrombocytopaenic Purpura
NR = Not Reported.

[+] CA = California; ID = Idaho; MA = Massachusetts; ME = Maine; MI = Michigan; MN = Minnesota; MO = Missouri; MT = Montana; NC = North Carolina; ND = North Dakota; NE = Nebraska; NV = Nevada; OR = Oregon; UT = Utah; WA = Washington; WI = Wisconsin

US data reproduced with the kind permission of Dr Patricia M Griffin from Infections of the Gastrointestinal Tract (in press), Ed: M J Blaser, H B Greenberg and R L Guerrant. Chapter 5.1 *E. coli* O157:H7 and Other Enterohaemorrhagic *E. coli*.[61]

TABLE 3.10

SELECTED GENERAL OUTBREAKS OF *E. COLI* O157:H7 INFECTION IN CANADA 1985-1993

Month and year	Setting	Cases	HUS[1]	Deaths[1]	Likely vehicle	Means of Identifying Likely Vehicle
September 1985	Nursing home	73	12	19	Cold sandwiches/person-to-person	E/M
April 1986	School	46	3	0	Raw milk	E/M
June 1986	Nursing home	8		2	Unknown	
June 1987	Nursing home	15		2	Raw beef	M
July 1987	Nursing home	9			Person-to-person	M
July 1987	Girl's camp	12			Unknown	
September 1987	Nursing home	4			Environment hose (sink)	M
December 1987	Family	2			Hamburger/cutlet	M
December 1987	Day-care centre	4			Unknown	
February 1988	Nursing home	7			Unknown	
July 1988	Nursing home	40		1	Unknown	
July-August 1988	Severely retarded young people's facility	30		1	Unknown	
August 1988	Camp	6			Unknown	
January 1989	Hospital	3			Unknown	
March 1989	Restaurant	4			Unknown	
July 1989	Nursing home	11			Unknown	
September 1989	Nursing home	8			Unknown	
August 1990	Nursing home	8			Unknown	
August 1990	Day-care centre	9			Unknown	
September 1990	Nursing home	7			Unknown	
June 1991	Community	98+	1+	2	Person-to-person	E/M
August 1991	Community	9			Ground beef	M
September 1991	Community	26	7	7	Ground beef	M
January 1992	Nursing home	4			Unknown	
August 1992	Community	6			Unknown	
July 1993	Community	12			Unknown	

E = epidemiological   M = microbiological   [1]Blank cells = not known or no cases.

Notes: 8 Canadians were associated with the Jack-in-the-Box restaurant chain outbreak in the USA in January 1993. In the period 1982 to 1993 a total of 62 general and 200 family outbreaks of *E. coli* O157:H7 infection were recorded in Canada.

Prepared by the National Reference Laboratory for Enteric Pathogens, Laboratory Centre for Disease Control, Health Canada.

Outbreaks and implicated sources of infection since 1982

3.39   From 1982 to 1993, 19 reported outbreaks of *E. coli* O157:H7 infection were investigated in the US (See Table 3.9). Outbreaks have occurred in schools, day-care centres, nursing homes, prisons and in the community. Outbreaks are usually detected because of a cluster of HUS or TTP cases often associated with an increase in the number of individuals hospitalised because of bloody diarrhoea. In the period 1982 to 1993, 62 general and 200 family outbreaks of *E. coli* O157:H7 infection were recorded in Canada. Table 3.10 provides information on selected outbreaks of *E. coli* O157:H7 infection in Canada from 1985 to 1993.

3.40   Most outbreaks have been associated with foods of bovine origin, particularly minced beef, often with evidence of inadequate cooking, (deficiencies in time/temperature combinations) so that all coliforms were not inactivated. In one exceptional outbreak, illness was associated with medium or rare roast beef and not recorded in those who ate the same beef well-done. Implicated meat vehicles are usually only slightly undercooked before ingestion rather than held at temperatures that would permit bacterial growth.[56] Human illness due to *E. coli* O157 has been linked to the consumption of minced beef since 1982 in the US,[62, 63] and with raw cows' milk since 1986.[64, 65]

3.41   From an analysis of Canadian outbreak information, 2 groups of people appear to be at higher risk, young children in day-care centres and the elderly in nursing homes. There were 45% of outbreaks which occurred in nursing homes, 15% in day-care centres and the rest, in the family and community.[66]

3.42   In a case-control study conducted during an epidemic of *E. coli* O157 in a remote community in northern Canada, 19 children with HUS were compared with 19 children with uncomplicated *E. coli* O157 gastroenteritis. Both of these groups were matched with 19 healthy controls. Undercooked ground meat and foods traditionally consumed by the community were not implicated as risk factors. The conclusion of the study was that extensive intrafamilial transmission had occurred.[67]

3.43   A large community outbreak occurred in Missouri between December 1989 and January 1990 from which a case-control study showed that no food was associated with illness but ill persons had drunk more municipal water than controls. *E. coli* O157 was not isolated from water samples but the number of cases decreased after an order to boil water and after chlorination of the water supply. Sewage contamination of the water supply during repairs to water mains is thought to have been the cause of the outbreak.[68]

3.44   A case-control study of an outbreak of diarrhoea and HUS in Massachusetts in 1991 indicated that illness was associated with drinking "unfermented apple cider". The term apple cider is used in the US to refer to apple juice. Most of the apples were "drops", collected from the ground and were not washed before using. The "apple cider" was not pasteurised and no preservative was added. Additional studies showed that *E. coli* O157 was able to survive in the refrigerated "apple cider" (pH < 4.0) for several days.[69]

3.45 An outbreak of *E. coli* O157 associated with mayonnaise occurred in 1993 [70] (see Table 3.9), and *E. coli* O157 has been shown to survive for a short time in mayonnaise stored at 25°C, and for much longer periods in mayonnaise-based sauces stored at refrigeration temperatures.[71]

3.46 *E. coli* O157 has been shown to survive for some time in manured soil. A first case in a small outbreak in Maine was a lacto-ovo-vegetarian whose diet consisted of vegetables from her garden which were fertilised with manure from her cow and calf.[72] Although faecal samples from both animals did not yield the pathogen, both had high antibodies to *E. coli* O157 LPS, and *E. coli* O157:H7 was isolated from manured soil in the garden. It should be borne in mind that manure from cattle may contain *E. coli* O157:H7 and care must be taken to avoiding contaminating crops such as salads and fruit when it is used as a fertilizer.

3.47 The range of sources implicated in studies of sporadic cases is similar to that for outbreaks i.e. undercooked meat (especially minced beef), raw cows' milk, untreated water, and person-to-person spread.[4, 73, 74]

US outbreaks in 1993

3.48 In January 1993, a large outbreak of *E. coli* O157:H7 was identified in Washington State. Smaller outbreaks in Nevada, California and Idaho were subsequently linked to the same vehicle, hamburgers consumed at multiple outlets of a single restaurant chain. A total of 732 patients were affected. Of these, 195 were hospitalised and 55 developed HUS or TTP; there were 4 deaths (Table 3.8). In Washington State there were 614 patients involved, of whom 491 were culture positive for Verocytotoxin producing *E. coli* O157:H7, and 11.8% of cases were determined to be secondary to a case who had contracted the disease via consumption of a contaminated hamburger. The median age of the patients was 7.5 years, 35 patients developed HUS and 3 died.[75, 76]

3.49 This important outbreak occurred during the time that the Working Group was collecting evidence. Laboratory diagnosis of infection, isolation from food, investigation of the source of the outbreak and subsequent control and prevention measures are all described in detail in Appendix 3.3.

3.50 In 1993, a small family outbreak of diarrhoea and bloody diarrhoea occurred in California where the vehicle of infection was traced to home-cooked hamburgers made from meat purchased from a local market. *E. coli* O157:H7 was isolated from leftover minced beef used to make the hamburgers and found to be the same 'phage type as the human isolate. It has been proposed that small outbreaks similar to the one described probably occur throughout the US but are not recognised.[77]

EPIDEMIOLOGY OF VTEC INFECTION IN EUROPEAN COUNTRIES OTHER THAN THE UK

WHO Surveillance Programme for control of foodborne infections and intoxications in Europe

3.51   In the WHO Fifth Report 1985-1989 published in 1992,[78] only nine out of thirty one participating countries mentioned *E. coli* in their reports and only one (Germany) of the nine specified a particular serogroup (0124).   However, one of the recommendations for the surveillance programme stated:

-   specific national surveys should be encouraged, particularly in relation to emerging and newly important diseases of possible foodborne origin, for example haemorrhagic colitis and haemorrhagic uraemic syndrome caused by Verocytotoxin-producing *E. coli* (eg. *E. coli* O157).

3.52   In December 1991, the WHO reported a consultation on "Shiga-like" toxin producing *E. coli*, with special emphasis on zoonotic aspects.

The purpose and scope was:

"- to review current diagnostic methods for detecting Shiga-like toxin producing *E. coli* (SLTEC) and their application to epidemiology. Discussions will be extended to elaborate simple and common methodologies for identifying SLTEC, including identification of the source of infection;

-   to review current epidemiology of outbreaks due to SLTEC in North America, Europe and other regions, and to identify the magnitude of their public health consequences, with particular emphasis on zoonotic aspects, including livestock production and food of animal origin;

-   to discuss and identify *in vitro* and *in vivo* methods for diagnosis and research on *E. coli* Shiga-like toxin (SLT)-production and other SLT pathogenic mechanisms; and

-   to review current progress on immunology of SLTEC infection and intoxication in man and animals. Discussions will be extended to strategies and possible methodologies for vaccine production. "

Following this consultation a Working Group was set up and has met several times in order to promote international co-operation.

Central European, multi-centre study

3.53   The German-speaking Working Group of Paediatric Nephrology organised a multi-centre study of HUS patients between August 1986 and April 1991. 147 patients were enrolled from 28 centres throughout the former East and West Germany, eastern France, northern Switzerland and Austria. Stool samples were received from 129 patients and serum samples from 144 patients. The frequency of VTEC involvement in childhood HUS was assessed by bacterial isolation, faecal toxin detection, cytotoxicity assays, VT neutralisation tests and immunoglobulin specific *E. coli* O157 LPS ELISA.

3.54   The majority of the patients (92%) in the study had diarrhoea positive HUS (D+HUS), the mean age of onset was 3.6 years and the male:female ratio was 1:15. In common with the seasonal frequency in the UK and US, there was a peak in July and August.

3.55   VTEC were identified in 19 out of 118 stool samples from D+HUS patients (16%). No VTEC were isolated from stool samples from D-HUS patients. *E. coli* O157, non-motile and H7 were the most frequently isolated serotypes, other serogroups identified were 022, 026, 055, and 0111. Free faecal Verocytotoxin was detected in 16 patients associated with the isolation of VTEC.

3.56   A fourfold increase in VT neutralisation titre was detected in 18% of D+HUS patients and elevated serum IgM and IgA to *E. coli* O157 LPS were detected in 83%.

3.57   It is notable from these results that although *E. coli* O157 was the most frequently isolated serogroup there was a high frequency of non-motile strains (6 out of 10). Many *E. coli* O157 of North American origin produce both VT1 and VT2 whereas a high proportion of strains from this study produced only VT2. The diagnostic value of serum neutralisation tests was questionable in the population tested while the serum IgM level to *E. coli* O157 LPS was found to be of more value.[79]

VTEC in France, Belgium and Italy

3.58   In a French multi-centre study covering a range of different geographical areas, 6 VTEC strains were isolated from the stools of 69 children suffering from HUS. All 6 strains were serotype O103:H2. This serotype is commonly associated with diarrhoea in rabbits. However, a study of the genetic properties of the human and rabbit strains eliminated the possibility of horizontal transmission as the strains were genetically distinct.[80]

3.59   More recently two clusters of HUS have been reported in France, neither of which were associated with *E. coli* O157. Ten cases with an average age of 6 years were reported in the winter of 1992 in an area north of Paris. VTEC O111 was isolated from 5 cases. Person-to-person transmission was suggested or exposure to a common unidentified food source. Another cluster of 3 cases of HUS occurred in the spring of 1992 in children of less than 2 years of age resulting in one death. VTEC were isolated from one case. All the children had eaten fromage frais made of raw goats' and cows' milk.[81]

3.60   The incidence of VTEC infections in patients attending the University Hospital in Brussels was estimated between October 1990 and September 1993 by detecting VTEC in stool specimens. The study showed that sporadic infections with VTEC were occurring, but the majority of cases were associated with non-O157 strains.[82]

Most patients suffered from uncomplicated diarrhoea, a few presented with HC or HUS.

3.61 A nationwide surveillance system for HUS was introduced in Italy in 1988. Up to December 1993 diagnosis of VTEC infection by microbiological and serological means was established in 80 patients. The detection of antibodies to the O157 lipopolysaccharide provided serologic evidence that O157 VTEC are the most prevalent VTEC involved in HUS in Italy.[83]

Information on VTEC from Germany, Denmark, Netherlands and Spain

3.62 The Working Group wrote to 24 Government institutions and research establishments in 11 EU countries for information on surveillance/research in relation to VTEC. The responses received are summarised in Appendix 3.4. The information received does not allow any confident statement to be made regarding the extent of either research or surveillance into VTEC in Europe.

Conclusions

3.63 Incompleteness of the available data on the incidence of HUS over time makes it difficult to assess if HUS caused by *E. coli* O157 is increasing, decreasing or remaining steady. **(C3.1)**

3.64 Even though the surveillance system in the UK is more comprehensive than comparative systems in the US and elsewhere in Europe, different criteria are used by laboratories to decide when to examine stools for *E. coli* O157. It is therefore difficult to state categorically if the increase in isolates is due to an increase in infection rate or an increase in ascertainment. Results of the laboratory diagnosis survey suggest an increase in ascertainment has occurred since 1989. Given that approximately half of patients do not present with bloody diarrhoea (paragraph 2.2), the presence of blood in the stools is not a logical selection criterion for the examination for O157 VTEC, and more effective surveillance of human infection will not be possible unless diagnostic/clinical laboratories examine all diarrhoeal stool specimens for *E. coli* O157. **(C3.2)**

3.65 There is incomplete information on sources, routes of transmission and socio-economic costs associated with O157 VTEC infection, and even less about non-O157 VTEC. **(C3.3)**

Recommendations

3.66 We recommend that the Government ensures that relevant clinical groups set up national prospective surveillance studies of HC, HUS and TTP in all age groups. **(R3.1)**

3.67 We recommend that all clinical laboratories routinely examine all diarrhoeal stool specimens for *E. coli* O157. **(R3.2)**

3.68 We recommend that the Government, in association with PHLS and Health Authorities, ensures that during outbreaks, case-control studies are undertaken to provide up-to-date knowledge about sources, routes of transmission, risk factors, and socio-economic costs associated with VTEC infection in the UK. **(R3.3)**

CHAPTER 4

VTEC IN FARM ANIMALS

WORKING GROUP ON VEROCYTOTOXIN PRODUCING *ESCHERICHIA COLI*

Introduction

4.1 Although *Escherichia coli* (*E. coli*) forms part of the normal commensal microflora of the gastro-intestinal tract of agricultural livestock, some strains are an important cause of diarrhoea, the disease syndromes they cause usually being referred to as colibacillosis. Enteric colibacillosis, associated with diarrhoea and toxaemia, is the commonest manifestation of *E. coli* disease seen in England and Wales,[84] occurring most frequently in calves, lambs and piglets 1-3 days old. Systemic colibacillosis is less common and is associated with invasive strains of the organism. *E. coli* is also known to be a cause of mastitis in adult cattle.

Verocytotoxin producing *E. coli* (VTEC) in animals

4.2 VTEC have been associated with animal disease. Experimental infections in calves have produced diarrhoea and the characteristic attaching and effacing lesions in the intestine resulting from bacterial attachment to the epithelium.[28, 29, 85, 86,] There have also been reports of naturally occurring VTEC associated diarrhoeal disease in cattle.[86, 87, 88, 89, 90, 91]

4.3 A study of *E. coli* isolated from diseased farm animals in England and Wales between 1986 and 1991 found that 2.8% of bovine isolates, 6.1% of ovine isolates and 4% of porcine isolates produced Verocytotoxins.[84] The porcine VTEC isolates were mainly of the serogroups O138, O139 and O141, which are commonly associated with oedema disease of pigs.* Some, however, were from cases of gastro-enteritis, though whether Verocytotoxin is involved in the pathogenesis of this condition is not known as some VTEC strains also produce enterotoxin. The fact that the highest percentage of VTEC strains occurred among the ovine isolates deserves further investigation as there is little information on the role of Verocytotoxin as a cause of disease of sheep.

4.4 VTEC have also been isolated from the gastro-intestinal tracts of healthy animals.[65, 92, 93, 94] In a study carried out in the USA, VTEC isolates were recovered from 8.4% of healthy dairy cows and 19.0% of dairy heifers and calves.[65] Similar results were obtained in a Canadian survey which indicated that farm infection rates ranged from 0-60% for cows and 0-100% for calves.[93] The VTEC isolates recovered in these studies came from a diversity of serogroups, some of which are known to be pathogenic for man suggesting that cattle might act as a reservoir for VTEC.

---

*Oedema disease of pigs is associated with VT2 producing *E. coli*, but the toxin is a variant and as such is known as VT2e (e = oedema). Strains causing oedema disease are not associated with human disease, although there is a report of an episode of human infection with a strain of *E. coli* producing the VT2e.[264]

VTEC in animal products

4.5 VTEC strains belonging to a variety of *E. coli* serogroups have been isolated from a range of foods, including beef and pork products [15, 95, 96] (see Chapter 6). However, the VTEC strains belonging to serogroups other than O157 are diverse in their properties, with production of Verocytotoxin as the only common attribute.[97] None of the VTEC strains isolated from a study of VTEC in raw beef products possessed the "*eae*" gene associated with the ability to cause attaching and effacing lesions involved in the intimate attachment of some VTEC and enteropathogenic *E. coli* strains.[15] This prompted the suggestion that detailed studies are required on non-O157 VTEC strains from human, animal and food sources to assess which strains possess factors necessary for human virulence. Until then, the importance of Verocytotoxin-producing strains of *E. coli* other than O157:H7 as a cause of foodborne disease in man will remain unclear.

VTEC of the serotype O157:H7 in animals

4.6 Outbreaks and sporadic cases of human haemorrhagic colitis caused by *E. coli* O157:H7 in North America [54, 62, 98, 99] and Great Britain,[47, 100, 101, 102] are linked to the consumption of undercooked minced beef and unpasteurised milk and attest to the importance of this organism as a cause of foodborne disease and the role of cattle as potential reservoir of infection (see Chapter 3).

4.7 Further evidence exists that foods of bovine origin could act as a potential, but not exclusive, source of human infection.[103] Examination of 2,415 bovine faecal samples in the period 1987-1993 yielded 96 strains of *E. coli* O157:H7, while over the same period of time *E. coli* O157:H7 was isolated from 63 sporadic, but unrelated cases of human haemorrhagic colitis and haemolytic uraemic syndrome in the same area. Of the 63 human strains, 59 (94%) were of types also isolated from cattle. In contrast, 39 bovine strains represented 29 types of *E. coli* O157 which had not been isolated from humans. Interestingly, these results contrast with those of Paros *et al.*[104] in the USA who reported that 90% of the human isolates they tested did not match bovine isolates.

Occurrence of *E. coli* O157:H7 in cattle

4.8 *E. coli* O157:H7 has been isolated from apparently healthy cattle, most commonly dairy calves, in the course of herd investigations linked to outbreaks of human infection in the United States.[64, 65, 98] The organism has also been recovered from cattle in the course of surveys unrelated to human infection in the USA, Canada, Germany and the UK.[65, 92, 101, 105] In a survey of more than 1,000 dairy herds in 28 states of the USA involving the examination of faeces samples from some 7,000 pre-weaned calves, *E. coli* O157:H7 was isolated from 25 calves in 19 herds.[106] In a follow up study, involving 50 previously *E. coli* O157 negative herds and 14 *E. coli* O157 positive herds, *E. coli* O157 positive calves were found in 11 of the previously negative herds and 7 of the previously positive herds. These results suggest that infection in herds may be transitory and cannot be defined by testing a few animals at one time. Positive animals ranged from 10 days to 8 months with weaned calves three times more likely to test positive than unweaned calves.

4.9   A study of 60 dairy herds, 25 cow/calf herds and 5 feedlots carried out in the USA suggested that while the between herd incidence may be high (8-16%) and peak in the summer months, the prevalence of infection within herds can be low and vary both between different ages of livestock (adult cows showing a lower prevalence (2%) than calves and heifers (10%)) and with time.[107, 108] Some attempt was made to identify risk factors associated with the occurrence of infection. Small herd size, use of computerised feeders and the spreading of animal manure on pastures were positively associated with the occurrence of infection in herds; feeding cotton seed was negatively associated.

4.10   Information on *E. coli* O157:H7 infections in cattle in the UK is limited. A survey of bovine faeces samples submitted to Veterinary Investigation Centres (VICs) in Scotland, begun in 1992, has resulted in the isolation of the organism from 14 of 5,237 samples examined. Twelve of the positive samples were from calves less than 2 months old. *E. coli* O157:H7 was not detected in faecal samples from 1,542 sheep, 515 pigs and 392 poultry nor in faecal samples from 1,271 animals of other species including dogs, cats, goats and horses.[109] *E. coli* O157 were also isolated from 84 of 2,103 (3.99%) cattle presented for slaughter at an abattoir in Sheffield during July and August 1992.[102] Traceback investigations showed that the farms of origin for 34 of the *E. coli* O157 positive animals were geographically diverse (Yorkshire, Worcestershire, Nottinghamshire, Shropshire) suggesting that infected herds may be more common than had previously been thought.

4.11   There is little evidence that *E. coli* O157:H7 causes clinical disease in cattle and little is known about the epidemiology of infection and the factors associated with its occurrence in cattle herds. *E. coli* O157:H7 was isolated from 3 calves suffering from colibacillosis in Argentina,[88] and though most of the isolates made from calves in the Scottish VIC survey came from animals with diarrhoea, other pathogens such as *Cryptosporidium* or rotavirus were also present and may have been responsible, wholly or in part, for clinical disease.

4.12   A longitudinal study of *E. coli* O157:H7 infection in a dairy herd considered to have been the source of a small outbreak of human infection caused by the consumption of unpasteurised milk (Chapman, unpublished observations) has provided some interesting insights into bovine infections with this organism. Commencing in July 1993, rectal swabs were taken from all the milking cows at fortnightly intervals while the animals were at grass and at fortnightly/monthly intervals following winter housing in November of that year. During this period, 29 cows, out of a total herd size of 130, were found to excrete *E. coli* O157:H7 on one or more occasions: on no occasion was there any evidence of clinical disease. All the cows were negative in the 4 weeks prior to housing but in the weeks immediately following housing in November, the organism was recovered from a small number of animals, until the end of December. Thereafter, there was no evidence of faecal excretion until early May 1994, just before the herd was turned out for summer grazing.

4.13   The herd was self contained, breeding its own replacement stock. When these were examined in August 1993, examination of faeces samples showed that 9/16 calves under 3 weeks of age, 18/26 in-calf heifers and 3/8 dry cows were excreting the organism. The heifers had grazed a field over which manure from the dairy cows had been spread in the previous 4 weeks, suggesting that this may have been the source of their infection.

4.14   *E. coli* O157:H7 had been isolated from unpasteurised milk produced on the farm but when individual fore and mid-stream milk samples were collected and examined from all 130 cows on 2 separate occasions, some of which were known to be excreting the organism in faeces, *E. coli* O157:H7 was isolated from only 1 fore-stream milk sample. These observations suggest that the organism was not being excreted in the milk and that the human incident may have resulted from external contamination.

Occurrence of *E. coli* O157:H7 on cattle carcases

4.15   Although *E. coli* O157:H7 has been isolated from minced beef, and contaminated minced beef has been identified as the source of human foodborne infections, there is little published evidence to demonstrate that the organism has been introduced into the food chain from infected cattle via contaminated carcases. As part of their study of *E. coli* O157:H7 in cattle slaughtered in a Sheffield abattoir, Chapman *et al.*[102] examined samples of meat excised (a), from the surfaces of carcases of animals known to be excreting *E. coli* O157:H7 in their faeces immediately prior to slaughter and (b), from the surfaces of carcases of animals, adjacent on the slaughter line and from which *E. coli* O157:H7 had not been isolated. *E. coli* O157:H7 were isolated from 7/23 (30.4%) carcases of animals from which the organism had previously been isolated from rectal contents and from 2/25 (8%) carcases of animals, adjacent on the production line, from which the organism had not previously been isolated. The latter may have resulted from cross contamination during the carcase dressing process though it is not without possibility that the animals were excreting *E. coli* O157:H7 in their faeces in numbers so low as to be undetectable.

4.16   Preliminary results from a survey of beef carcases in the USA have revealed that *E. coli* O157:H7 was present on 0.2% of 2,081 randomly selected beef carcases examined over a 12 month period in 1992/93.[204] It is believed that similar surveys are currently taking place in Australia and New Zealand, as well as in the UK (see paragraph 4.22).

Red meat slaughtering

4.17   Carcases contaminated during the slaughtering and dressing process represent an important route by which pathogenic organisms such as *E. coli* O157:H7 can enter the food chain. The state of cleanliness of the animals and the skill and care exercised in the slaughter, dressing and evisceration processes play a significant part in the initial transfer of organisms from the hide and gastro-intestinal contents to the carcase surface. In this respect, the practice of rodding and bunging, which involves sealing the oesophagus and anus in cattle and sheep, can reduce the risk during evisceration. Thereafter, various factors such as rate of throughput, carcase washing etc. will contribute to the spread of contamination and affect the final microbiological load, while chilling and freezing will prevent the growth of the organisms that remain. Further opportunities for contamination will occur during the subsequent boning and cutting operations and any other process to which the meat might be subjected to before it reaches the consumer. In this respect, there is no reason to believe that the factors contributing to carcase contamination are in any way different for *E. coli* O157:H7 as compared with other enteropathogens such as *Salmonella* or *Campylobacter*.

The Committee on the Microbiological Safety of Food (Richmond Committee)

4.18   Red meat production was examined by the Committee on the Microbiological Safety of Food, chaired by Sir Mark Richmond.[110] The Richmond Committee emphasised the need for all those in the early stages of the red meat production chain to pass on a product in which microbiological contamination was kept to a practical minimum, and considered it vital that working conditions should be such as to enable operatives to do their work with due care to minimise the risk of carcases being contaminated. They concluded that high standards of hygiene could be achieved in red meat production if all concerned were fully aware of the microbiological risks and the steps that could be taken to minimise them. This applied to all stages of production, from the farm via the slaughterhouse/cutting plant to packaging and processing operations, and at all levels - from slaughterhouse workers being aware of the basic principles of personal hygiene to the design and selection of equipment. To this end, the Committee placed considerable emphasis on the recruitment and training of all levels of staff involved.

4.19   In their stage by stage consideration of the production chain, the Committee pointed out that farmers could contribute to food safety by producing healthy, clean animals for slaughter and minimising stress during transport so as to reduce the number of micro-organisms being introduced into the abattoir. In this respect, abattoir managers were recommended to pay farmers a premium to take account of cleanliness of animals as one component of quality. On-farm health records were also considered to be of potential use to those inspecting meat at slaughterhouses and it was thought that developments in electronic tagging might allow meat inspectors to identify an animal's farm of origin thereby allowing prompt access to health records and the transmission of post mortem data back to farmers.

4.20   The inadvertent introduction of microbiological contamination into the carcase or onto the carcase surface from the skin or hide via operator hands or implements were recognised as critical points in the slaughtering process and the Committee recommended the use of freshly sanitised knives for bleeding and questioned the continuing need for the practice of pithing. Rupture of the gastro-intestinal tract and spillage of its contents during evisceration were also seen as a prime source of carcase contamination and the Committee considered there should be greater awareness of the risks so that with adequate time, proper supervision and care, hygienic removal of the tract could be achieved. They further recommended industry to adopt the practice of tying and bagging the anus and sealing the oesophagus at its entrance to the rumen prior to its removal so as to minimise these risks.

4.21 The Committee considered that those designing slaughter equipment (which traditionally had speed of operation rather than hygiene as a priority) should make ease of cleaning a priority. Equipment in slaughterhouses and cutting plants which comes into repeated contact with meat should be regularly cleaned and disinfected. The high speeds of modern slaughterhouse equipment operation resulting in an increased microbiological hazard was a recurring theme in the Committee's analysis and led to a recommendation that slaughterhouse operatives and managers should be aware of the need to minimise contamination and the steps that should be taken to achieve this.

4.22 Finally, the Committee stressed the important contribution that microbiological monitoring could make to the HACCP approach, which they commended for slaughterhouses as for all other stages of food production. Its regular application to key equipment and to the carcase at the critical points in the slaughtering process would establish "normal" microbial levels in a given plant and thus provide a valuable early indication when there was a breakdown in hygiene arrangements which needed attention. Monitoring should also be used to check the effectiveness of cleansing and disinfection. The Committee recommended that the Steering Group on the Microbiological Safety of Food (SGMSF) consider how arrangements could best be made for work on microbiological monitoring to be taken forward. In this regard it should be noted that a national survey of *E. coli* O157:H7 contamination on beef carcases leaving abattoirs in the UK is currently being undertaken by the Steering Group and is due to be completed in August 1995.

European and national legislation on meat and meat products

4.23 With the completion of the Single European Market, the European Union now has a major role in determining law on food safety. Since the Richmond Committee published Part II of its Report in 1991, a number of Directives have been adopted establishing harmonised measures for the hygienic production of fresh meat throughout all Member States. Principle among these is Council Directive 91/497/EEC [111] amending Directive 64/433/EEC [112] which lays down health conditions for the production and placing on the market of fresh meat, which in Great Britain has been implemented through the Fresh Meat (Hygiene and Inspection) Regulations 1995.[263]

4.24 Under these Regulations, all slaughterhouses, cutting premises, cold stores and farmed game processing facilities must be licensed by the Government after 1 January 1993, licenses being issued only if the premises comply with prescribed requirements regarding their construction, layout, equipment and hygienic operation. Many of the recommendations made by the Richmond Committee are reflected in the Regulations particularly as regards the cleansing and disinfection of equipment and instruments that come into contact with fresh meat, and the ante and post mortem inspection of animals.

4.25 The Regulations also lay down detailed rules regarding the slaughter and dressing processes, including the removal of gastro-intestinal tracts, aimed at minimising carcase contamination. An official veterinary surgeon (OVS) must be appointed for each licensed premises, as must sufficient inspectors to carry out the functions specified in the Regulations under the supervision and responsibility of the OVS. The OVS and appointed inspectors have the power to require the detention or prohibit the slaughter of any animal which in their opinion is so dirty that it is likely to prevent hygienic dressing operations.

4.26   While the Regulations do not include general provisions regarding the identification of animals, all fresh meat (both whole carcases, parts of carcases and offals) which is passed as fit for human consumption must be marked with a 'health mark' which must contain the approval number of the abattoir/cutting plant premises. Meat must be chilled and transported at temperatures of not more than $+7°C$; $+3°C$ for offal and $-12°C$ for frozen fresh meat.

4.27   Council Directive 91/497/EEC requires licensed operators to carry out microbiological checks of utensils, fittings and machinery at all stages of production and, if necessary, of products. However, the nature of these checks, their frequency, the sampling methods and methods to be employed for sample examination have still to be agreed at Community level. No microbiological checks are therefore included in the Regulations.

4.28   Council Directive 92/5/EEC,[113] amending and updating Council Directive 77/99/EEC, [114] lays down harmonised rules for the manufacture, storage, handling and distribution of meat products up to the point they are supplied to the final consumer. It also specifies the structural and hygienic requirements for premises engaged in manufacturing and rewrapping meat products. The Directive has been implemented in Great Britain by the Meat Products (Hygiene) Regulations 1994.[115] These Regulations do not include any specific microbiological criteria. However, they do require the operator of the production establishment or rewrapping centre to take samples for analysis for the purpose of checking cleansing and disinfection methods, and for checking compliance with the standards laid down in the Directive. When laboratory examination or any other information reveals there to be a serious public health risk, the competent authority must be informed. In the event of an immediate risk to human health, the operator must withdraw the affected product from the market and arrange suitable disposal.

4.29   Council Directive 88/657/EEC [116] lays down requirements for the production of minced meat and meat preparations despatched to other Member States but does not apply to domestic trade. It has been implemented in Great Britain on an administrative basis pending implementation of Single Market rules. Directive 88/657 contains prescriptive temperature controls and microbiological criteria adopted in the main to control minced meat which is consumed raw. It will be replaced by Directive 94/65/EC [117] which is due to come into force from 1 January 1996. This sets down detailed conditions for intra-Community trade in minced meat and meat preparations with Member States able to derogate from certain provisions for products traded in their national markets. Production of minced meat and meat preparations may only take place in premises approved by the competent authority and the operators of such premises are required to adopt a HACCP approach, monitor the quality and microbiological status of both the raw material and finished products entering and leaving their premises, and take action on the basis of criteria laid down in the Directive.

Carcase decontamination

4.30 Even under the best hygienic conditions achievable, it is probably impossible to ensure that animal carcases are totally free of micro-organisms, most of which will comprise non-pathogenic spoilage organisms. Interest is therefore increasing in the use of sanitizing agents such as acetic or lactic acids, trisodium phosphate, hot water washes and hyperchlorinated water for terminal carcase decontamination. However, it has to be emphasised that such processing aids must be regarded only as a supplement and not a replacement for preventive hygiene measures. While early research on the use of such processing aids shows promise, existing European legislation prohibits the use of any substance other than potable water for carcase washing.[118]

Conclusions

4.31 Verocytotoxin producing strains of *E. coli* are known to be a cause of enteric disease, especially in pigs and cattle. **(C4.1)**

4.32 The recovery of Verocytotoxin producing strains of *E. coli* other than *E. coli* O157:H7 from the gastro-intestinal tracts of healthy agricultural livestock and from a range of foods of animal origin, indicates that farm animals can act as a reservoir of human infection. However, the contribution non-O157 VTEC make to human food-borne disease remains unclear pending detailed studies to assess which strains possess the factors necessary for human virulence. **(C4.2)**

4.33 *E. coli* O157:H7 is known to occur in agricultural livestock, often without causing disease. The epidemiology of *E. coli* O157:H7 infection in cattle is poorly understood as are the factors associated with its occurrence. There is evidence that infection may be transitory. **(C4.3)**

4.34 *E. coli* O157:H7 has been recovered from the carcase surfaces of cattle slaughtered in the UK and North America, and undercooked minced beef and milk are considered to be potential sources of human infection. **(C4.4)**

4.35 Even under the best hygienic conditions achievable, it is probably impossible to ensure that animal carcases are totally free of micro-organisms, most of which will comprise non-pathogenic spoilage organisms. Nevertheless, all possible measures should be taken to minimise the extent and level of microbiological contamination of carcases. **(C4.5)**

4.36 We endorse the views expressed by the Richmond Committee on the need for all those involved in the early stages of the red meat production chain to pass on a product in which microbiological contamination is kept to a practical minimum and that high standards of hygiene can be achieved in red meat production if all concerned are fully aware of the microbiological risks and the steps that can be taken to minimise them. **(C4.6)**

4.37 We welcome the SGMSF's national survey of *E. coli* O157:H7 contamination on beef carcases leaving abattoirs in the UK. **(C4.7)**

Recommendations

4.38 We further endorse the Richmond Committee's recommendation that a dedicated programme of training and continuing in-job development is required in order to create an expert cadre of staff committed to high standards of hygienic slaughterhouse practice. **(R4.1)**

4.39 We recommend that Government funds research in the following areas:

- to establish the incidence/prevalence of *E. coli* O157:H7 in UK cattle/cattle herds and other agricultural livestock;

- to improve understanding of the epidemiology of *E. coli* O157:H7 infections in agricultural livestock and identify the husbandry and other factors contributing to herd infection and control; and

- the effectiveness of processing aids, such as carcase washes, in further reducing the microbiological load on carcases. **(R4.2)**

CHAPTER 5

LABORATORY METHODS FOR THE DETECTION OF VTEC IN CLINICAL SAMPLES AND FOOD

Introduction

5.1   The methods used to provide evidence of VTEC infection can be divided into three categories. These are the isolation of VTEC including *E. coli* O157, demonstration of specific Verocytotoxin and the presence of antibodies to *E. coli* O157 lipopolysaccharide (LPS) or the LPS of other VTEC serogroups. Some of these methods can be performed in most laboratories while other techniques are usually limited to specialized or reference laboratories.

Isolation from clinical samples

5.2   Laboratories usually screen selected specimens, from cases of bloody diarrhoea and HUS, for the presence of O157 VTEC. In clinical laboratories faeces are plated on solid media and currently MacConkey agar containing sorbitol is most often employed. With very few exceptions O157 VTEC do not ferment sorbitol unlike most other *E. coli*. The colonies that appear as non-sorbitol fermenting are tested by agglutination for *E. coli* O157 antigens. Improvements in the selectivity of media have been described (see Appendix 4.1, Table A.4.1). It is essential that all presumptive *E. coli* O157 isolates are confirmed using both biochemical and serological techniques.

Isolation from foods and environmental samples

5.3   The methods for the isolation of O157 VTEC from foods and environmental samples need to be as sensitive as possible since the number of organisms present may be very low. Standard procedures for isolation of *E. coli* from foods include growth at 44°C. However, this is not appropriate for O157 VTEC since these organisms grow very poorly at 44°C and it is emphasised that lower temperatures should be used.

5.4   Methods for the isolation of O157 VTEC from foods and environmental samples usually require growth in liquid media for enrichment of the organism. Several different media have been reported (Appendix 4.1). After growth in liquid media, *E. coli* O157 can be selectively enriched by use of magnetic beads coated with an O157 antibody. This is followed by plating on solid media such as sorbitol MacConkey agar and subsequent confirmation by agglutination with specific antisera. Alternative methods have been developed after enrichment in liquid media and these have been aimed primarily at screening in the food industry and other large scale surveillance studies. Such methods include an ELISA kit specific for O157 VTEC and a blot ELISA (Appendix 4.1).

Detection of Verocytotoxin and VT genes

5.5   VTEC may be detected by the demonstration of Verocytotoxin or the presence of genes encoding VT. This approach detects all VTEC including those of serogroup O157. Bacterial cultures or faecal extracts can be examined for a cytotoxic effect on Vero monkey kidney cells grown in tissue culture (see Appendix 4.1). In order to demonstrate the specificity of any toxic effects neutralization experiments with specific antisera to Verocytotoxins need to be performed. Although these tests are very sensitive they require specialised facilities and specific antisera are not commercially available at present.

5.6   The presence of VT genes can be detected by specific DNA probes in hybridization experiments or by amplification using primers from the VT gene sequences in a polymerase chain reaction (PCR). Non-radioactively labelled probes for VT genes have been developed and should enable DNA hybridization to be applied in a wide range of laboratories. This approach can be used for clinical as well as food and environmental samples. These methods detect all VTEC and not just *E. coli* O157.

Sub-typing VTEC

5.7   VTEC belonging to serogroups other than O157 should be serotyped with antisera against the currently recognised 173 O antigens and 55 H antigens. For VTEC of serogroup O157, 'phage typing has been particularly useful in epidemiological investigations. The scheme first developed in Canada now recognizes over 80 types. Other techniques that are being applied for the differentiation of VTEC are VT sub-typing by DNA probes or PCR, plasmid analysis and a range of other molecular techniques based on the analysis of the genomic DNA (see Appendix 4.2).

Serodiagnosis

5.8   Evidence for infection by *E. coli* O157 can also be obtained by examining sera. Patients with a known O157 VTEC infection develop an increase in the level of antibodies to the LPS of *E. coli* O157. Tests have been developed for the detection of these antibodies (see Appendix 4.3) and have proved to be very useful in providing evidence of infection when culture methods have been negative especially late in the clinical disease. In contrast, antibodies to the Verocytotoxins have been rarely detected and such investigations are not recommended for serodiagnosis.

Conclusions

5.9   Solid media with improved selectivity for the isolation of O157 VTEC have been described. Sorbitol-fermenting O157 VTEC strains such as those reported in Germany would not be detected. **(C5.1)**

5.10   Most laboratories only test for O157 VTEC as tests able to detect all VTEC are not suitable for clinical laboratories. The clinical and epidemiological importance of non-O157 VTEC cannot be fully assessed at present. **(C5.2)**

5.11 VTEC isolates should be sent to a reference laboratory for confirmation and sub-typing in order to maximise epidemiological information. **(C5.3)**

5.12 Tests for antibodies to *E. coli* O157 LPS can often provide evidence of infection when culture methods are negative and particularly late in the disease. **(C5.4)**

5.13 Methods for the isolation of O157 VTEC from foods and environmental samples need to be able to detect very low levels, and also to be suitable for use in the food industry. Significant improvements have resulted from use of liquid enrichment and development of methods such as immunomagnetic separation for *E. coli* O157. **(C5.5)**

Recommendations

5.14 We recommend that the Government funds research into the following areas:

- the development and evaluation of different solid media for O157 VTEC;

- rapid methods to detect VTEC of all serogroups and Verocytotoxin in food and clinical material; and

- the development of methods for improved sub-typing of VTEC and particularly O157 VTEC. **(R5.1)**

5.15 We recommend that the Government and industry fund the evaluation of conventional and rapid methods for the examination of foods and environmental samples for O157 VTEC. **(R5.2)**

5.16 We recommend that the Government continues to support reference laboratory facilities for O157 VTEC and non-O157 VTEC, in order to maximise epidemiological information. **(R5.3)**

CHAPTER 6

VTEC IN FOOD AND PREVENTION AND CONTROL MEASURES

Introduction

6.1   Control and prevention of VTEC infection will ultimately depend on reducing the numbers of VTEC in the whole food chain. Achievement of this goal will be greatly helped by an increase in our understanding of the epidemiology, physiology and pathogenicity of VTEC, and by the application of HACCP principles to food production and storage. In this chapter the incidence, growth and survival characteristics of VTEC in food are considered to form the basis for recommending practical measures that can be taken by the food industry and consumers to minimise the risk of VTEC infection.

Occurrence in food

6.2   The reported occurrence of VTEC, including *E. coli* O157:H7, in foods is shown in Table 6.1. Undoubtedly, the variability in the reported occurrence is partly due to differences in the sensitivity of the methods used (see Chapter 5).

6.3   In a study of raw beef products in the UK, VTEC was detected in 13-22% of samples, and *E. coli* O157:H7 non-VT producing strains in 1.6% of samples.[119] In another study in the UK no VTEC were detected in raw chicken, but 25% of samples of raw pork sausage were found to be positive.[96] Surveys done mainly in North America have reported the detection of VTEC and *E. coli* O157 in a variety of raw meats (Table 6.1).

6.4   A large survey of milk, dairy and associated samples in the UK failed to detect *E. coli* O157. In this study a number of different detection methods were used, but the efficiency of recovery was deemed to be poor using artificially-contaminated samples.[120]

6.5   Various foods have been implicated in several countries as potential vehicles in incidents or outbreaks of VTEC infection (see Chapter 3). Such foods include minced meat, burgers, roast beef, turkey roll, raw (unpasteurised) cows' milk, yoghurt, mayonnaise, fromage frais (made of raw goats' and cows' milk), vegetables, "unfermented apple cider" (apple juice), water, milk from a heat-treated supply, and cheese made from raw cows' milk.

6.6   In the UK, O157 VTEC was detected for the first time in food in 1993, using the immunomagnetic separation (IMS) technique (see Chapter 5). A small outbreak in England was associated with the consumption of raw cows' milk, and O157 VTEC was isolated from a milk sample taken from the cow.[47] Later in 1993, O157 VTEC was isolated from a raw beefburger obtained from a retail source linked to a small community outbreak in Wales.[15]

6.7 In Scotland, O157 VTEC was isolated for the first time in 1994, using an IMS technique, from a heat-treated milk supply that was implicated in the largest milkborne outbreak to date. The outbreak was associated with the consumption of milk from a local dairy. Many environmental samples were taken in the dairy and a pipe that carried milk from the pasteurisation apparatus to the bottling machine and a discarded bottle machine rubber yielded O157 VTEC indistinguishable from the human isolates.[50]

6.8 In another Scottish outbreak of O157 VTEC infection in 1994, cheese made from raw cows' milk was shown to be the vehicle of infection. However, surface contamination of the cheese during storage, in the retail chain, or by symptomatic cases could not be ruled out. Descriptive epidemiology supported such contamination rather than a failure of the cheese-making process (personal communication Dr J Curnow, Grampian Health Board).

Factors affecting growth and survival in foods

6.9 VTEC may be present in raw foods, so an understanding of the factors affecting growth, survival and elimination is essential for control. As *E. coli* O157:H7 appears to have a low infectious dose (see Chapters 2 and 3), growth of the bacterium in food may not be a prerequisite for disease. Therefore, its ability to survive in adverse conditions may be significant. The majority of data available relates specifically to *E. coli* O157:H7; other VTEC may not necessarily behave in the same manner. From the currently available information, *E. coli* O157:H7 appears to grow, survive and die in similar circumstances to other foodborne pathogens, with the possible exception of its acid tolerance.

6.10 Within the UK Predictive Food Microbiology Programme (Food MicroModel), the effects of temperature, pH, salt (sodium chloride) and carbon dioxide on the growth, survival and thermal inactivation of *E. coli* O157:H7 have been studied and models are available.[127] The range of conditions for the models is given in Table 6.2.

Temperature

6.11 Growth rates increase with rising temperature through the chill to warm range, until the optimum is reached. The optimum is reported to be 37°C and the maximum is 45°C.[128]

TABLE 6.1

EXAMINATION OF FOODS FOR THE PRESENCE OF VTEC AND *E. COLI* O157:H7 - INFORMATION FROM FOOD SURVEYS

	COUNTRY	FOOD	DETECTION (% positives)	METHOD	COMMENT	REFERENCE
(i) VTEC	UK	Raw minced beef	17/134 (13%)	1, 2	a, b	Willshaw et al.[119]
		Raw beef sausage	9/52 (17%)			
		Raw beefburger	27/124 (22%)			
	UK	Raw chicken	0/71 (0%)	1	a	Smith et al.[96]
		Raw pork sausage	46/184 (25%)			
	UK	Milk and dairy samples	0/1146 (0%)	4, 5		Neaves et al.[120]
	USA	Raw beef	14/60 (23%)	1	a	Samadpour et al.[121]
		Raw pork	9/51 (18%)			
		Raw lamb	10/21 (48%)			
		Raw veal	5/8 (63%)			
		Raw chicken	4/33 (12%)			
		Raw turkey	1/15 (7%)			
		Raw fish	6/62 (10%)			
		Raw shellfish	2/44 (5%)			
	Canada	Raw beef	82/225 (36%)	1	a	Read et al.[95]
		Raw pork	25/235 (11%)			
		Raw chicken	0/200 (0%)			
	Thailand	Raw beef	8/93 (8.6%)	1	a	Suthienkul et al.[122]
		Raw chicken	1/107 (0.9%)			
		Raw pork	1/111 (0.9%)			
		Raw vegetables	0/130 (0%)			

64

TABLE 6.1 - *Continued*

	COUNTRY	FOOD	DETECTION (% positives)	METHOD	COMMENT	REFERENCE
(ii) *E. coli* O157:H7	USA	Raw beef Raw veal kidney Raw chicken	2/1668 (0.1%) 9/4953 (0.2%) 0/3977 (0%)			Griffin and Tauxe[56]
	USA	Raw beef Raw pork Raw poultry Raw lamb	6/164 (3.7%) 2/264 (1.5%) 4/263 (1.5%) 4/205 (2.0%)	2, 3		Doyle and Schoeni[123]
	USA	Raw beef Raw milk	3/107 (2.8%) 11/115 (10%)	4		Padhye and Doyle[124]
	USA	Cheese	0/50 (0%)	5		Bowen and Henning[125]
	Canada	Raw ground beef	4/165 (2.4%)			Sekla *et al.*[126]

Methods

1, DNA probes for VTEC
2, DNA probes for O157:H7
3, Filtration
4, ELISA
5, Petrifilm

Comments

a, none of the VTEC were confirmed as *E. coli* O157:H7
b, some O157:H7 isolated, not VT producing

65

TABLE 6.2

LIMITS OF PREDICTION FOR GROWTH, SURVIVAL AND THERMAL DEATH OF *E. COLI* O157:H7 FROM FOOD MICROMODEL

(i)	Growth/survival model	
	Temperature	10-30°C
	pH	4.5-7.0
	NaC1 (w/v)	0.0-6.5%
	* A_w	0.96-1.00
	CO_2	0-80%
(ii)	Thermal Death	
	Temperature	54.5-64.5°C
	pH	4.2-9.8
	NaC1 (w/v)	0.0-8.5%
	* A_w	0.946-1.0

The limits given above for this model should not be taken as definitive for growth, survival or death for this micro-organism.

* A_w is based on salt as the solute.

<u>Freezing</u>

6.12 Relatively little information is available on the effects of freezing on *E. coli* O157:H7, but it has been reported that this bacterium survives freezing at -80°C in ground beef patties, and that little change in numbers occurred during 9 months storage at -20°C.[128] In another study, only 9 of 23 previously positive samples were viable after frozen storage for 1 year.[129] As with other bacteria, the degree of injury and death caused by freezing is likely to be dependent on the rate of freezing, the temperature of frozen storage and the rate of thawing.

<u>Chill temperatures</u>

6.13 It has been reported that growth may occur in laboratory media at 6.5-7.2°C when other conditions are favourable for growth,[130, 131, 132] and growth in foods has been reported at temperatures as low as 8°C in "unfermented apple cider" (see para 3.44), and at 12°C in lettuce.[133, 134] Whilst growth has not been reported at temperatures below 6.5°C, this bacterium may survive at such temperatures for considerable periods. Good refrigeration below 5°C will prevent growth of *E. coli* O157:H7. Under adverse pH and salt conditions that do not permit growth, chill storage may enhance the opportunity for survival.[133]

<u>High temperatures</u>

6.14 The effects of temperature, pH and salt (sodium chloride) on the heat resistance of *E. coli* O157:H7 may be predicted using Food MicroModel [127] (Table 6.2). In general, the heat resistance of bacteria is affected by the interaction of temperature, pH and salt. A study was made of the heat resistance of *E. coli* O157:H7 in pork and chicken homogenate over the temperature range 54-64°C.[135] The highest D-value obtained in chicken homogenate at 64°C was 0.46 minutes; the z-value was 7.3°C.

6.15 In a Canadian study, the pasteurisation of milk* (72°C for 16.2 seconds) has been reported to eliminate over 10,000 *E. coli* O157:H7 per ml.[136] Although *E. coli* O157:H7 grew during manufacture of cottage cheese, it was destroyed by the processing temperatures used to cook the curd (57°C for 90 minutes).[137]

6.16 As with other bacteria, the reported heat resistance of *E. coli* O157:H7 may be affected by a number of factors and the heat process may have to be designed accordingly. The heat resistance may be increased if the bacterium is grown anaerobically rather than aerobically.[138] It was established that VTEC strains were more resistant to heat when they were in the stationary phase (i.e. at the end of their rapid growth phase).[139] In common with most bacteria, the heat resistance in foods is often greater than in media. Furthermore, it was reported that resistance was greater in fatty rather than lean beef.[140] Within the UK Predictive Food Microbiology Programme, it has been noted that the type of humectant may affect the heat

---

*In the UK the pasteurisation of milk requires 71.7°C for 15 seconds or equivalent time/temperature combinations.

resistance, with *E. coli* O157:H7 being more resistant in sugar solution rather than in salt solution at the same water activity value. Finally, heat shocking of *E. coli* O157:H7 (i.e. prior exposure to mild heat) at 42°C for 5 minutes has been reported to increase the subsequent heat resistance at 55°C by a factor of 1.5 to 2.1.[138] From the available information, it may be concluded that heat resistance of *E. coli* O157:H7 is similar to that of *Salmonella*.

Water activity

6.17   Little published information is available on the effects of water activity or humectants on the growth of VTEC. A study showed that *E. coli* O157:H7 grows well at sodium chloride concentrations up to 2.5% w/v and may grow at 6.5% w/v (A_w approximately 0.97) when other factors are favourable for growth.[141] Sodium chloride concentrations in excess of 8.5% w/v inhibit growth. The growth of *E. coli* O157:H7 was inhibited at sodium chloride concentrations of 8% w/v and above at 37°C, but by 4-6% w/v at 10°C depending upon growth medium.[142] The effect of other humectants (e.g. sugars) on the growth of VTEC is less clear at this time.

Acid tolerance

6.18   An early indication of the significance of the acid tolerance of these organisms occurred in 1991, when a case control study demonstrated a strong epidemiological association between locally produced live yoghurt and infection.[48] Further evidence came in 1993 from an outbreak of HC in the US, that was attributable to the consumption of "unfermented apple cider" a product equivalent to unprocessed apple juice in the UK. It has subsequently been shown that *E. coli* O157:H7 could be recovered from inoculated, "unfermented apple cider" (apple juice) for up to 2 or 3 days when stored at 25°C, but for up to 31 days when stored at 8°C.[183] Enhanced survival in acid conditions at low temperatures (8°C), compared with room temperature, has also been claimed with mayonnaise (pH 3.8) in the US where there was an outbreak associated with the product.[70, 71]

6.19   The minimum pH for growth is considered to be pH 4.5 (using hydrochloric acid) when other conditions are favourable.[141] Under less favourable conditions, reduced temperature or decreased water activity, the minimum pH for growth may be higher (i.e. less acidic). The minimum pH is also affected by the type of acid present. Acetic acid was found to be more inhibitory than lactic acid and both were more effective than hydrochloric acid.[131] This has also been reported for other pathogens such as *Salmonella*.

6.20   As the pH of a product decreases (i.e. it becomes more acidic), the rate of inactivation of *E. coli* O157:H7 increases.[143] The fermentation processes applied to many cultured products cannot guarantee the elimination of *E. coli* O157:H7 from foods and additional controls may be necessary.[137, 141] Overall, this bacterium is able to tolerate acidic conditions better than *Salmonella*.[144]

Gamma irradiation

6.21   Studies on the effects of irradiation on *E. coli* O157:H7 in mechanically de-boned chicken meat and minced beef revealed a complex interaction between temperature, atmosphere and irradiation dose, but have led to the conclusion that a moderate dose of 1.5-2.5 kGy would be adequate to eliminate this organism from finely minced meats.[145, 146]

Other factors

6.22   Although there is little information available about the effect of chemical preservatives, sorbate and benzoate have been shown to be capable of limiting growth of *E. coli* O157:H7 and in some cases may increase the rate of non-thermal inactivation.[133, 147] The effectiveness of these preservatives is highly dependent on the pH of the food, temperature of storage and salt content.

6.23   There is scant information in the public domain on the effectiveness of food grade detergents and sanitisers on freely suspended and attached *E. coli* O157:H7 in food environments. This bacterium has been isolated from food contact surfaces.[50]

6.24   Aerobic storage tends to enhance growth of *E. coli* O157:H7 compared with anaerobic conditions, but the differences are generally minimal, indicating that this bacterium is well adapted to both situations.[148] Modified atmosphere packaging of *E. coli* O157:H7 under conditions typical of fresh vegetable produce had little effect on the growth or survival characteristics of this bacterium.[134]

Prevention and control of VTEC in foods

6.25   The fail-safe option for the control of VTEC in foods is to accept that these organisms may be present on or in a low percentage of raw meats including mechanically recovered meat, raw milk and raw vegetables despite efforts to prevent this happening. The prevention of disease caused by the organisms must be assured by the good hygiene and manufacturing practices of the primary producers, manufacturers, retailers, food service establishments and consumers. Many of the following paragraphs reiterate comments made in our Interim Report on *Campylobacter* which are also relevant to VTEC.[149]

HACCP

6.26   The Hazard Analysis Critical Control Point (HACCP) system is well established as one of the best means of ensuring the safety of foods.[150, 151, 152, 153] The application of this type of system, therefore, will provide a structured approach to the prevention or limitation of the occurrence of VTEC in the food supply.

6.27 Knowledge of the occurrence, growth and survival characteristics of organisms in food can be used to analyse the potential hazards in an operation and to decide which are critical to consumer safety. These Critical Control Points (CCPs) are monitored and remedial action is taken if conditions at the CCP approach defined limits. In the UK, a HACCP based approach to the control of hazards in foods has been promoted by Government and adopted by many sectors of the industry. The Government published a leaflet entitled "Practical Food Safety for Businesses" in 1991, which was sent to environmental health departments for dissemination to food businesses in the UK. The leaflet was designed as an introduction to HACCP principles and how to adopt them.

6.28 One of the strengths of the HACCP approach is that it can be applied throughout the whole food chain, from the primary production and purchase of raw materials to the serving of the food for final consumption. Although there are a number of sectors in the food chain, there are only a few types of operation involved: primary purchase, production, manufacture, storage, cooking and cooling. The preventative measures that need to be taken during these operations to eliminate or reduce VTEC apply equally to businesses and consumers as appropriate and each party has a responsibility to ensure that they are implemented appropriately.

Raw materials

6.29 One major objective should be to eliminate, or reduce, the levels of VTEC in raw materials as much as possible. This will reduce the risk of these micro-organisms being present in food in sufficient numbers to infect consumers should the production processes be inadequate to eliminate them.

6.30 If VTEC are present on any raw material, then they must be eliminated at some point in the production process, otherwise they present a hazard when the food is consumed. The typical control options open to the food industry at purchase are for buyers to undertake hygiene inspections of the supplier's premises and establish raw material specifications, which will help ensure the quality of the raw material.

- Raw beefburgers and other minced meat products

6.31 The US Government has recently introduced the mandatory labelling of raw meat products, with written and pictorial instructions for the consumer on safe handling, cooking and storage (See A.3.3.20). As the mincing process allows any organisms that might be present on the surface of the raw meat to be distributed throughout the product, beefburgers and other minced meat products pose a greater hazard than intact joints of meat. Instructions on labels could help to ensure correct cooking of raw minced beef and minced beef products in the UK (e.g. beefburgers and sausages), an important CCP for the safe preparation of these foods. As the Government's ability to prescribe labelling is limited by EU law, industry could introduce voluntary labelling. This would accord with industry's general obligation to provide instructions necessary for the use of pre-packed food.

6.32 Vendors (i.e. manufacturers, retailers and wholesalers) of raw beefburgers have the responsibility of ensuring that the minced meat has come from a reputable source and has been handled in a hygienic manner. This should include correct temperature control to prevent growth of VTEC and measures to prevent cross-contamination. This applies equally well to frozen and to chilled beefburgers.

- Raw (unpasteurised) milk and associated products

6.33 A number of outbreaks of *E. coli* O157:H7 in the UK and North America have been associated with the consumption of raw cows' milk (see Chapter 3). Outbreaks of infection caused by *Campylobacter* and *Salmonella* have also been associated with the consumption of raw cows' milk.[154] The Government has twice in recent years proposed that pasteurisation of cows' milk should be obligatory. This proposal has not been implemented because public consultation showed a strong consumer demand for raw cows' milk among a section of the population. However, the Government has introduced various controls which have restricted the availability and consumption of raw cows' milk. One of these controls is that raw cows' milk must be labelled: "This milk has not been heat-treated and may therefore contain organisms harmful to health".

6.34 It is clear that raw cows' milk may transmit O157 VTEC in addition to other pathogens, and because VTEC had not been found in raw cows' milk in the UK when the Government last considered banning its sale, we have decided to recommend that the Government should reconsider its position. Our decision was influenced by:

a)   two outbreaks of O157 VTEC disease in the UK associated with raw or contaminated pasteurised cows' milk (see Chapter 3);

b)   the severity of the illness (see Chapter 2);

c)   the low infectious dose of O157 VTEC (see Chapters 2 and 3);

d)   the fact that raw cows' milk could be consumed by vulnerable groups including children; and

e)   the fact that raw cows' milk is consumed without any further processing to eliminate the organism.

6.35 We understand that cream made from raw cows' milk may be sold at farmgate and in retail outlets in England, Wales and Northern Ireland. It must, however, come from an approved establishment and the words: "made from raw milk" must appear on the label. Although there is no direct evidence as yet linking this product to VTEC infection, we do not consider that the separation process involved in the production of cream would necessarily remove any O157 VTEC if present in the original raw cows' milk. We consider that cream made from raw cows' milk should be subject to the same regulations as raw cows' milk (see Appendix 5 for information on EC and UK legislation on unpasteurised cows' milk and cream).

6.36 We considered cheeses made from raw milk and concluded that, as for cream made from raw milk, there is no direct evidence as yet linking them to VTEC infection in the UK, although in an outbreak of O157 VTEC infection in Scotland in 1994, cheese made from raw cows' milk was shown to be the vehicle of infection (see paragraph 6.8). However, we note that VTEC is relatively acid tolerant (see paragraphs 6.18-6.20) and we are satisfied that the acidification that occurs during the cheese making process cannot be relied upon to kill VTEC. In the meantime, more information is needed on the occurrence of VTEC in cheeses made from raw milk, and consumers should be informed when a cheese is made from raw milk.

Storage of raw materials, intermediate and finished goods

6.37 The conditions of storage for raw materials, intermediate and finished goods, should be such as to prevent contamination of the materials with VTEC and other pathogens. Storage times and temperatures should ensure that growth does not occur.

Heating

6.38 Heating is one operation that can be used to eliminate VTEC consistently and as such is one of the major CCPs in the food chain. Current experience suggests that, as far as food is concerned, minced beef and milk seem to be the most common vehicles for VTEC infection. Both of these commodities rely on heating as their main CCP.

6.39 It is important that heating equipment, including microwave ovens, must be capable of consistently achieving an effective time/temperature combination in every part of the food. The cooking process must be monitored and remedial action taken if the time/temperature combination is not achieved. Further details are given in the leaflet "Safer Cooked Meat Production Guidelines",[155] and for consumers, in the "Cooking Food" section of the Foodsense Food Safety Leaflet.[156]

- Pasteurised milk

6.40 There is a well established Critical Control Point (CCP) for milk processing in the pasteurisation processes which are clearly defined in existing legislation. By applying HACCP principles to milk pasteurisation plants and ensuring adherence to well recognised good manufacturing practices, pasteurised milk should pose no threat to human health [110] (see also paragraphs 6.7 and 6.58).

- Beefburgers - thermal death of VTEC

6.41 A considerable amount of research has shown that VTEC are similar to other vegetative pathogens in their sensitivity to destruction by heat in a variety of circumstances (see paragraphs 6.14-6.16). However, recognising the critical importance of cooking of beefburgers to eliminate VTEC, MAFF commissioned research at the Campden and Chorleywood Food Research Association (CCFRA) to investigate the way that heat destroys the organism if it is present in beefburgers.

6.42   Two strains of VTEC associated with human infection in the UK were inoculated at various levels into a range of minced beefburgers which were then heated to a variety of temperatures chosen to reflect those generally used in catering or in the home. From these experiments, the thermal death kinetics of VTEC in beefburgers were determined using standard microbiological methods. The standard way of expressing the heat sensitivity of an organism is to calculate the 6D-value, which is the combination of time and temperature needed to eliminate 1,000,000 cells per gram of food. The results so far indicate that the 6D-value for VTEC in beefburgers is equivalent to 70°C for 2 minutes. This appears to eliminate VTEC. Equivalent values to 70°C for 2 minutes are shown in Table 6.3. These values are greater than the USDA Regulations published in 1993 which were supported by the FDA Food Code published early in 1994.[157, 158]

6.43   The CCFRA study showed also that at 70°C for 2 minutes or equivalent values, the juices of the burger ran clear and there were no pink bits inside. This is in line with the Chief Medical Officer's advice in 1991 that beefburgers should be cooked until the juices run clear, and there are no pink bits inside. However, it must be stressed that the burgers used in the study contained only beef and that burgers containing other ingredients such as cured meats might not turn brown during cooking. Given that this visual assessment of cooking is often the only practical check available to caterers and consumers that the burgers have been adequately cooked, more research is needed to ascertain the factors affecting the colour of beefburgers of all types under all normal conditions of cooking and handling. For example, a recent study has found that the colour of the meat in beefburgers is not always a reliable indicator of safe cooking.[159] It should be stressed that this advice is meant to apply only to minced meat products such as beefburgers and is not intended to apply to whole joints of meat, as VTEC would not be expected to be present in the centre of intact joints of meat.

- Beefburgers - retailers

6.44   Vendors of raw beefburgers should ensure that the burger is supplied with cooking instructions adequate to destroy VTEC by the time and temperature equivalents printed in Table 6.3 and/or the instructions "cook thoroughly until the juices run clear and there are no pink bits inside". Cooking instructions should take into account factors such as whether the burger is frozen or chilled, the thickness and formulation of the burger and the prescribed method of cooking. Purchasers of raw beefburgers should, as far as is practicable, ascertain that the above conditions have been met. They should also ensure that the product is stored at the appropriate temperature in such a way that it is protected from cross-contamination, and that it cannot cross-contaminate other foods, particularly ready-to-eat foods such as lettuce, other salad vegetables and mayonnaise. Consumers should follow the cooking instructions provided by the vendor.

73

TABLE 6.3

EQUIVALENT HEAT TREATMENTS

Temperature °C	Time
60	45 minutes
65	10 minutes
70	2 minutes
75	30 seconds
80	6 seconds

Source: Reproduced from "Safer Cooked Meat Production Guidelines".[155]

6.45   Vendors of cooked beefburgers (i.e. caterers) should ensure that the burger has been cooked according to the instructions given in section 6.44. They should consider the potential for undercooked burgers to cause VTEC associated disease and should not provide customers with undercooked burgers, or if specifically requested to do so, should remind the customer of the potential hazard. Consumers should ensure that the burgers they purchase are cooked thoroughly by checking that they are brown throughout and that the juices, if any, run clear. Consumers should also avoid premises where cooked and raw meat are not separated, and where assistants are seen to handle raw food and then touch cooked food without washing their hands thoroughly in-between. Consumers should inform their local Environmental Health Department when these unhygienic practices are encountered. Consumers should follow the advice given in the "Shopping for Food" section of the Foodsense Food Safety Leaflet.[156]

6.46   Persons preparing instructions for the cooking of beefburgers or cooking beefburgers must pay particular attention to the following factors:

-    The formulation of the beefburger (if known) - Different ingredients may affect the final colour of the product. For example, the inclusion of cured meats or curing salts might result in a burger that remains pink in the middle, even after prolonged cooking.

-    The thickness of the burger - Thicker burgers may require longer cooking than thinner burgers to ensure that they are properly cooked throughout.

-    Defrosting - It is vital to ensure that frozen beefburgers are properly defrosted prior to cooking or that if they are intended to be cooked from frozen, then the cooking instructions take this into account. This is particularly important in catering situations. For example, a recent (unpublished) survey conducted by 6 local authority Environmental Health Departments (in southwest London) found that out of 150 catering premises surveyed, 142 (95%) purchased raw burgers in the frozen state. Of these 142 businesses, 77 (54%) fully defrosted burgers before cooking them, 27 (19%) partially defrosted the burgers before cooking them, while the remaining 38 (27%) cooked them from frozen. It is particularly important, therefore, that catering operations are set up in such a way that a sudden rush of customers does not result in frozen beefburgers being cooked in an operation designed to work with partially or fully defrosted burgers, otherwise not all the burgers may be adequately cooked.

- Methods of cooking

6.47   During our visits to caterers and manufacturers of beefburgers, we observed a number of different techniques in use for cooking burgers. Regardless of the technique used, it is critical that the operation can consistently achieve 70°C for 2 minutes or equivalent in all parts of every burger.

6.48   Given that cooking is so critical to consumer safety, we believe that the cooking process must be monitored and remedial action taken if the burgers are not properly cooked. The monitoring can be as simple as checking that the juices run clear, or it may involve measuring the centre temperature of the burger. Either way, if the correct cook is not achieved, then the burger should either be cooked further or discarded and the cooking process re-evaluated. If temperature probes are used then they must be properly and regularly maintained and calibrated.

Cross-contamination

6.49   As a consequence of the low infectious dose of *E. coli* O157:H7, cross-contamination is a major concern. Although there are many ways in which cross-contamination can occur, it falls into two broad categories: direct and indirect. Direct cross-contamination is where the cause of the contamination directly contacts the food, e.g. a piece of raw meat touching a ready-to-eat food. Indirect cross-contamination is where the transfer of micro-organisms is via another material such as a knife or a dishcloth. Indirect cross-contamination can sometimes occur via a chain of events, such as raw meat to chopping board, chopping board to dishcloth, dishcloth to plate, plate to food. The potential for cross-contamination of both domestic and industrial equipment emphasises the need for regular and thorough cleaning.

6.50   General advice on avoiding cross-contamination is available from a number of sources such as the "Safer Cooked Meat Production Guidelines",[155] "Guidelines on Cook-Chill and Cook-Freeze Catering Systems",[160] "Assured Safe Catering",[153] and for consumers from "Food Safety".[156] Common guidance for industry, much of which applies equally to the avoidance of cross-contamination in the domestic kitchen, was outlined in the ACMSF report on *Campylobacter*[149] which is also relevant to VTEC, as follows:

-   Raw foods must be handled in a separate area from cooked foods unless their processing is separated by time and the area effectively cleaned in between;

-   Hands should be washed before any food is handled and especially after handling raw meat;

-   Separate utensils, including thermometer probes, should be used for cooked and raw foods (the same utensils can be used if effectively cleaned in between);

-   All cleaning equipment, including dishcloths and kitchen towels, should be sanitised thoroughly before using in areas in which cooked foods will be handled;

-   Raw foods, used utensils or surfaces likely to cause contamination, should never be allowed to come into contact with cooked foods;

- Where possible, separate staff should be used in high risk/high care (cooked foods) and low risk/low care (raw foods) areas;

- Separate refrigerators should be used for cooked and raw foods. If this is not possible then raw foods should not be stored above cooked foods; and

- Only potable water should be used for processing foods and for cleaning.

Food hygiene training and information

6.51 As it is unlikely that the numbers of VTEC entering the food chain will ever be reduced to zero, possible sources of infection will continue to be present in the commercial and domestic kitchen. VTEC infections could be significantly reduced if there was a better understanding of the need to avoid cross-contamination and to cook food properly in order to kill any organisms that may be present. Broadly the advice that we would offer to the two primary groups involved are:

(i) Commercial food handlers - Focus training on methods for the safe and hygienic handling of food. The Draft Food Safety (General Food Hygiene) Regulations 1994 include a broad requirement for food businesses to supervise, instruct and/or train their staff in food hygiene in a way commensurate with their tasks in the preparation or handling of food.

(ii) Consumers - Maintain chill temperatures, proper storage, adequate cooking and the hygienic preparation of foods. A large volume of food safety information is available to the public, much of which has been provided by the major supermarket chains in the form of booklets. The Government has also produced a series of "Foodsense" leaflets.[156] Thorough cooking and the avoidance of cross-contamination are of particular importance in avoiding infection by VTEC, and particular attention should be directed towards informing consumers of these matters.

Conclusions

6.52 *E. coli* O157:H7 survives well in frozen storage and freezing cannot be relied upon to kill the bacterial cells. **(C6.1)**

6.53 Although the heat resistance of *E. coli* O157:H7 is similar to *Salmonella*, additional information on the heat resistance of *E. coli* O157:H7 is required to provide definitive process recommendations for all relevant foods. **(C6.2)**

6.54 The ability of *E. coli* O157:H7 to tolerate acidic conditions appears to be greater than that of *Salmonella*. **(C6.3)**

6.55 The use of irradiation could be an effective measure to control VTEC. **(C6.4)**

6.56 HACCP is a well-established system for industry to identify and control potential contamination by VTEC. **(C6.5)**

6.57 Outbreaks of *E. coli* O157:H7 associated with the consumption of raw cows' milk have resulted in severe illness and occasionally deaths in young children and the elderly. **(C6.6)**

6.58 VTEC contamination in pasteurised milk supply has occurred and could follow either a breakdown in good hygiene practices or post-pasteurisation contamination or a failure in the pasteurisation process. **(C6.7)**

6.59 The extent of contamination of raw meats, raw cows' milk, cream made from raw cows' milk, and cheese made from raw milk from cows and other species is unknown. **(C6.8)**

6.60 There is a need for more research into the survival of VTEC in the food processing environment and methods for its control. **(C6.9)**

6.61 The effect of differences in the formulation of beefburgers may affect the colour changes in the meat during heating. **(C6.10)**

6.62 It is important that consumers are clearly informed of the recommended practices for handling and cooking of raw minced meat and minced meat products including beefburgers. **(C6.11)**

Recommendations

6.63 We recommend that all relevant sectors of the food industry adopt a HACCP-based approach to prevent survival of or contamination by VTEC. **(R6.1)**

6.64 We strongly urge the Government to reconsider its position concerning a ban on the sale of raw cows' milk in England, Wales and Northern Ireland. In the meantime, vulnerable groups in particular should be advised by the Government's Chief Medical Officer not to consume it, and the labelling of raw cows' milk should be altered accordingly. **(R6.2)**

6.65 We recommend that industry ensures that the pasteurisation of milk and milk products is carefully controlled and that post-pasteurisation contamination is avoided. **(R6.3)**

6.66 We recommend that industry label cheese made from raw milk from cows and other species so that consumers can identify it. **(R6.4)**

6.67 We recommend that industry label raw minced beef and minced beef products with appropriate handling and cooking instructions. **(R6.5)**

6.68 We endorse the Chief Medical Officer's advice that burgers should be cooked until the juices run clear, and there are no pink bits inside. This advice should be reconsidered when results of the research recommended into the relationship between the formulation and colour of cooked minced meat products, the colour of juices, and the temperature achieved and the survival of VTEC are available. **(R6.6)**

6.69   We endorse the Government's advice to cook minced beef and minced beef products including beefburgers to a minimum internal temperature of 70°C for 2 minutes or equivalent. This advice should be reviewed when the results of the relevant research mentioned in R6.10 are known. **(R6.7)**

6.70   We recommend that industry should ensure that the cooking instructions supplied with beefburgers should be capable of achieving an internal temperature of 70°C for 2 mins (or equivalent), so that the burger's juices run clear, and there are no pink bits inside. This advice should be reviewed when the results of the relevant research mentioned in R6.10 are known. **(R6.8)**

6.71   We recommend that persons preparing instructions for the cooking of beefburgers or cooking beefburgers must pay particular attention to the formulation of the burger; its thickness; the methods of defrosting and cooking used, and should monitor the cooking process, taking remedial action when necessary. **(R6.9)**

6.72   We recommend that the Government and industry fund research and surveillance into:-

-    the prevalence of O157 VTEC in raw meats, raw cows' milk, cream made from raw cows' milk, and raw milk cheeses;

-    the nature and extent of the acid resistance of VTEC;

-    the relationship between the formulation and colour of cooked minced meat products, the colour of juices, and the temperature achieved and the survival of VTEC; and

-    the effect of sanitisers/disinfectants on the survival of VTEC. **(R6.10)**

CHAPTER 7

CONCLUSIONS AND RECOMMENDATIONS

Chapter 2: Clinical Spectrum and Disease

Conclusions

C2.1 VTEC infection in man may arise from ingestion of a small number of organisms. The most common presentation of symptomatic VTEC infection is diarrhoea, which may be bloody (HC) in approximately 50% of patients. (2.20)

C2.2 A small proportion (2-15%) of those with VTEC infection may develop haemolytic uraemic syndrome (HUS); this progression is most likely to occur in children under 5 years and the elderly. Deaths, though rare, are more often seen in adults with VTEC related illness than in other age groups. (2.21)

C2.3 The efficacy of antibiotic treatment in modifying the disease is unclear. (2.22)

C2.4 Damage to vascular endothelial cells in many tissues by VTs is an important consequence of VTEC infection. (2.23)

C2.5 The attachment to intestinal cells by most, but not all, VTEC strains is likely to be mediated by specific adhesins (which have yet to be determined); attachment is followed by tissue damage. (2.24)

Recommendations

R2.1 We recommend that all those involved in managing outbreaks make use of the available guidance on the public health measures to control VTEC infection. (2.25)

R2.2 We recommend that the Government should consider funding research in the following areas:

- factors affecting the outcome of VTEC diarrhoeal illness, including the role of protective factors (age, sex, blood group) in progression to HUS;

- effectiveness of clinical intervention in treating cases of VTEC infection and HUS; in particular, more needs to be known about the efficacy of antibiotics in affecting carriage, spread of infection and outcome of infection;

- characterisation of the adhesins of VTEC strains, including the minority that do not produce the characteristic (attaching and effacing) lesions;

- *in vitro* methods for demonstration and detection of pathogenicity determinants to aid laboratory diagnosis; and

- the relationship between VTEC diversity in VT and adhesin production and clinical disease. (2.26)

Chapter 3: Epidemiology of VTEC Infections in Humans

Conclusions

C3.1 Incompleteness of the available data on the incidence of HUS over time makes it difficult to assess if HUS caused by *E. coli* O157 is increasing, decreasing or remaining steady. (3.63)

C3.2 Even though the surveillance system in the UK is more comprehensive than comparative systems in the US and elsewhere in Europe, different criteria are used by laboratories to decide when to examine stools for *E. coli* O157. It is therefore difficult to state categorically if the increase in isolates is due to an increase in infection rate or an increase in ascertainment. Results of the laboratory diagnosis survey suggest an increase in ascertainment has occurred since 1989. Given that approximately half of patients do not present with bloody diarrhoea (paragraph 2.2), the presence of blood in the stools is not a logical selection criterion for the examination for O157 VTEC, and more effective surveillance of human infection will not be possible unless diagnostic/clinical laboratories examine all diarrhoeal stool specimens for *E. coli* O157. (3.64)

C3.3 There is incomplete information on sources, routes of transmission and socio-economic costs associated with O157 VTEC infection, and even less about non-O157 VTEC. (3.65)

Recommendations

R3.1 We recommend that the Government ensures that relevant clinical groups set up national prospective surveillance studies of HC, HUS and TTP in all age groups. (3.66)

R3.2 We recommend that all clinical laboratories routinely examine all diarrhoeal stool specimens for *E. coli* O157. (3.67)

R3.3 We recommend that the Government, in association with PHLS and Health Authorities, ensures that during outbreaks, case-control studies are undertaken to provide up-to-date knowledge about sources, routes of transmission, risk factors, and socio-economic costs associated with VTEC infection in the UK. (3.68)

Chapter 4: VTEC in Animals

Conclusions

C4.1 Verocytotoxin producing strains of *E. coli* are known to be a cause of enteric disease, especially in pigs and cattle. (4.31)

C4.2 The recovery of Verocytotoxin producing strains of *E. coli* other than *E. coli* O157:H7 from the gastro-intestinal tracts of healthy agricultural livestock and from a range of foods of animal origin, indicates that farm animals can act as a reservoir of human infection. However, the contribution non-O157 VTEC make to human food-borne disease remains unclear pending detailed studies to assess which strains possess the factors necessary for human virulence. (4.32)

C4.3 *E. coli* O157:H7 is known to occur in agricultural livestock, often without causing disease. The epidemiology of *E. coli* O157:H7 infection in cattle is poorly understood as are the factors associated with its occurrence. There is evidence that infection may be transitory. (4.33)

C4.4 *E. coli* O157:H7 has been recovered from the carcase surfaces of cattle slaughtered in the UK and North America, and undercooked minced beef and milk are considered to be potential sources of human infection. (4.34)

C4.5 Even under the best hygienic conditions achievable, it is probably impossible to ensure that animal carcases are totally free of micro-organisms, most of which will comprise non-pathogenic spoilage organisms. Nevertheless, all possible measures should be taken to minimise the extent and level of microbiological contamination of carcases. (4.35)

C4.6 We endorse the views expressed by the Richmond Committee on the need for all those involved in the early stages of the red meat production chain to pass on a product in which microbiological contamination is kept to a practical minimum and that high standards of hygiene can be achieved in red meat production if all concerned are fully aware of the microbiological risks and the steps that can be taken to minimise them. (4.36)

C4.7 We welcome the SGMSF's national survey of *E. coli* O157:H7 contamination on beef carcases leaving abattoirs in the UK. (4.37)

Recommendations

R4.1 We further endorse the Richmond Committee's recommendation that a dedicated programme of training and continuing in-job development is required in order to create an expert cadre of staff committed to high standards of hygienic slaughterhouse practice. (4.38)

R4.2 We recommend that Government funds research in the following areas:

- to establish the incidence/prevalence of *E. coli* O157:H7 in UK cattle/cattle herds and other agricultural livestock;

- to improve understanding of the epidemiology of *E. coli* O157:H7 infections in agricultural livestock and identify the husbandry and other factors contributing to herd infection and control; and

-   the effectiveness of processing aids, such as carcase washes, in further reducing the microbiological load on carcases. (4.39)

Chapter 5: Laboratory Methods for the Detection of VTEC in Clinical Samples and Food

Conclusions

C5.1 Solid media with improved selectivity for the isolation of O157 VTEC have been described. Sorbitol-fermenting O157 VTEC strains such as those reported in Germany would not be detected. (5.9)

C5.2 Most laboratories only test for O157 VTEC as tests able to detect all VTEC are not suitable for clinical laboratories. The clinical and epidemiological importance of non-O157 VTEC cannot be fully assessed at present. (5.10)

C5.3 VTEC isolates should be sent to a reference laboratory for confirmation and sub-typing in order to maximise epidemiological information. (5.11)

C5.4 Tests for antibodies to *E. coli* O157 LPS can often provide evidence of infection when culture methods are negative and particularly late in the disease. (5.12)

C5.5 Methods for the isolation of O157 VTEC from foods and environmental samples need to be able to detect very low levels, and also to be suitable for use in the food industry. Significant improvements have resulted from use of liquid enrichment and development of methods such as immunomagnetic separation for *E. coli* O157. (5.13)

Recommendations

R5.1 We recommend that the Government funds research into the following areas:

-   the development and evaluation of different solid media for O157 VTEC;

-   rapid methods to detect VTEC of all serogroups and Verocytotoxin in food and clinical material; and

-   the development of methods for improved sub-typing of VTEC and particularly O157 VTEC. (5.14)

R5.2 We recommend that the Government and industry fund the evaluation of conventional and rapid methods for the examination of foods and environmental samples for O157 VTEC. (5.15)

R5.3 We recommend that the Government continues to support reference laboratory facilities for O157 VTEC and non-O157 VTEC, in order to maximise epidemiological information. (5.16)

Chapter 6: VTEC in Food and Prevention and Control Measures

Conclusions

C6.1 *E. coli* O157:H7 survives well in frozen storage and freezing cannot be relied upon to kill the bacterial cells. (6.52)

C6.2 Although the heat resistance of *E. coli* O157:H7 is similar to *Salmonella*, additional information on the heat resistance of *E. coli* O157:H7 is required to provide definitive process recommendations for all relevant foods. (6.53)

C6.3 The ability of *E. coli* O157:H7 to tolerate acidic conditions appears to be greater than that of *Salmonella*. (6.54)

C6.4 The use of irradiation could be an effective measure to control VTEC. (6.55)

C6.5 HACCP is a well-established system for industry to identify and control potential contamination by VTEC. (6.56)

C6.6 Outbreaks of *E. coli* O157:H7 associated with the consumption of raw cows' milk have resulted in severe illness and occasionally deaths in young children and the elderly. (6.57)

C6.7 VTEC contamination in pasteurised milk supply has occurred and could follow either a breakdown in good hygiene practices or post-pasteurisation contamination or a failure in the pasteurisation process. (6.58)

C6.8 The extent of contamination of raw meats, raw cows' milk, cream made from raw cows' milk, and cheese made from raw milk from cows and other species is unknown. (6.59)

C6.9 There is a need for more research into the survival of VTEC in the food process environment and methods for its control. (6.60)

C6.10 The effect of differences in the formulation of beefburgers may affect the colour changes in the meat during heating. (6.61)

C6.11 It is important that consumers are clearly informed of the recommended practices for handling and cooking of raw minced meat and minced meat products including beefburgers. (6.62)

Recommendations

R6.1 We recommend that all relevant sectors of the food industry adopt a HACCP-based approach to prevent survival of or contamination by VTEC. (6.63)

R6.2 We strongly urge the Government to reconsider its position concerning a ban on the sale of raw cows' milk in England, Wales and Northern Ireland. In the meantime, vulnerable groups in particular should be advised by the Government's Chief Medical Officer not to consume it, and the labelling of raw cows' milk should be altered accordingly. (6.64)

R6.3 We recommend that industry ensures that the pasteurisation of milk and milk products is carefully controlled and that post-pasteurisation contamination is avoided. (6.65)

R6.4 We recommend that industry label cheese made from raw milk from cows and other species so that consumers can identify it. (6.66)

R6.5 We recommend that industry label raw minced beef and minced beef products with appropriate handling and cooking instructions. (6.67)

R6.6 We endorse the Chief Medical Officer's advice that burgers should be cooked until the juices run clear, and there are no pink bits inside. This advice should be reconsidered when results of the research recommended into the relationship between the formulation and colour of cooked minced meat products, the colour of juices, and the temperature achieved and the survival of VTEC are available. (6.68)

R6.7 We endorse the Government's advice to cook minced beef and minced beef products including beefburgers to a minimum internal temperature of 70°C for 2 minutes or equivalent. This advice should be reviewed when the results of the relevant research mentioned in R6.10 are known. (6.69)

R6.8 We recommend that industry should ensure that the cooking instructions supplied with beefburgers should be capable of achieving an internal temperature of 70°C for 2 minutes (or equivalent), so that the burger's juices run clear, and there are no pink bits inside. This advice should be reviewed when the results of the relevant research mentioned in R6.10 are known. (6.70)

R6.9 We recommend that persons preparing instructions for the cooking of beefburgers or cooking beefburgers must pay particular attention to the formulation of the burger; its thickness; the methods of defrosting and cooking used, and should monitor the cooking process, taking remedial action when necessary. (6.71)

R6.10 We recommend that the Government and industry fund research and surveillance into:-

-    the prevalence of O157 VTEC in raw meats, raw cows' milk, cream made from raw cows' milk and raw milk cheeses;

-       the nature and extent of the acid resistance of VTEC;

-       the relationship between the formulation and colour of cooked minced meat products, the colour of juices, and the temperature achieved and the survival of VTEC; and

-       the effect of sanitisers/disinfectants on the survival of VTEC. (6.72)

GLOSSARY

This glossary is intended as an aid to the reading of the main text and is not intended to be definitive.

AETIOLOGY
The study of the causation of disease.

AGGLUTINATION
The clumping together of antigens by antibodies so that a visible agglutinate is formed.

ANAEMIA
The lack of red cells, or of their haemoglobin (the oxygen-carrying substance) in blood.

ANAEROBICALLY
In the absence or near absence of oxygen.

ANTIBODY
A protein formed in direct response to the introduction into an individual of an antigen. Antibodies can combine with their specific antigens e.g. to neutralise toxins or destroy bacteria.

ANTIGEN
A substance which elicits an immune response when introduced into an individual.

ANTISERUM
A solution which contains antibodies.

ASYMPTOMATIC INFECTION
An infection with a micro-organism where the person infected does not suffer any resulting symptoms or disease.

BACTERICIDAL
Able to kill at least some types of bacteria.

BACTERIOPHAGE TYPING
A method for distinguishing varieties of bacteria ('phage types) within a particular species on the basis of their susceptibilities to a range of bacteriophages (bacterial viruses).

BACTERIUM
A microscopic organism with a rigid cell wall; often unicellular and multiplying by splitting in two.

BIOTYPING
A method for distinguishing varieties of bacteria by metabolic and/or physiological properties.

CASE
A person in the population identified as having a particular disease.

CASE-CONTROL STUDY
An epidemiological study in which the characteristics of persons with disease (e.g. their food histories) are compared with a matched control group of persons without the disease or infection.

COLONISATION
The phenomenon of a community of micro-organisms becoming established in a certain environment (especially in the intestinal tract of humans or animals) without necessarily giving risc to disease.

COLONY IMMUNOBLOTTING
A serological technique for detecting specific micro-organisms.

COMMENSAL
An organism which derives benefit from living in close physical association with another organism, the host, which derives neither benefit nor harm from its relationship with the commensal.

CULTURE MEDIUM
A liquid or solid medium which is capable of supporting the growth of micro-organisms.

DNA HYBRIDISATION
The matching of a DNA fragment (e.g. a DNA probe) to a target DNA sequence.

DNA PROBE
A DNA fragment that has been labelled with a marker to indicate when DNA hybridisation has occurred.

D-VALUE
The time required at a given temperature to reduce the number of viable cells or spores of a given micro-organism to 10% of the initial number, usually quoted in minutes.

ELISA (Enzyme-Linked Immunosorbent Assay)
A serological test which uses enzyme reactions as indicators.

ENDOTHELIAL CELLS
Cells which form the layer (the endothelium) lining the inner surface of blood and lymph vessels and the heart.

ENTEROTOXIN
A toxin that causes gastroenteritis.

EPIDEMIOLOGY
The study of factors affecting health and disease in populations and the application of this study to the control and prevention of disease.

EPITHELIAL CELLS
Cells which form the layer (the epithelium) lining the inner surface of the intestines.

FLAGELLUM
An long hair-like appendage on the surface of the cell whose movement is used for cellular locomotion.

FLAGELLAR ANTIGEN
The antigen on the flagella known as the "H" antigen.

GRAM NEGATIVE
A reaction of a staining procedure used as an initial step in the identification of bacteria.

HAEMOLYTIC URAEMIC SYNDROME (HUS)
A clinical condition which may arise from a variety of causes, and is characterised by anaemia and kidney failure.

HAEMORRHAGIC COLITIS (HC)
Inflammation and bleeding from the large bowel that may be caused by an infectious agent.

HUMECTANT
A substance which absorbs moisture.

IgA, IgG, IgM
Different types of immunoglobulin (antibody) found in body fluids.

IMMUNOCOMPROMISED
An individual who is unable to mount a normal immune response.

IMMUNOGLOBULINS
A class of proteins which are antibodies and found in body fluids.

IMMUNOLOGICAL TESTS
Tests based on antigen-antibody reactions.

IMMUNOMAGNETIC SEPARATION (IMS)
A technique for isolating a particular microorganism using magnetic beads coated with antibodies to that organism.

INCIDENCE
The proportion of the population that contracts a disease during a particular period of time.

INCUBATION PERIOD
The time interval between the initial entry of a pathogen into a host, and the appearance of the first symptoms of disease.

INDEX CASE
The first case in an outbreak of infectious disease.

INFECTIOUS DOSE
The amount of infectious material, e.g. number of bacteria, necessary to produce an infection.

IN VITRO

Literally "In glass" ie. in a test tube, plate etc. Used to describe biological processes made to happen in laboratory apparatus, outside a living organism

ISOLATE

Bacterial growth originating from a particular sample.

LIPOPOLYSACCHARIDE (LPS)

That part of the outer membrane of Gram negative bacterial cells which functions as "O" antigens.

MASTITIS

Inflammation of the mammary gland.

MICROFLORA

The microbial population of an area such as the gastro-intestinal tract.

MOTILE STRAINS

Bacterial strains which can move independently.

OUTBREAK

Two or more cases of disease linked to a common source.

PASTEURISATION

A form of heat treatment that kills vegetative pathogens and spoilage bacteria in milk and other foods.

PATHOGEN

Any biological agent that can cause disease.

PATHOGENESIS

The manner in which a disease develops.

PATHOGENICITY

Ability to behave as a pathogen.

pH

An index used as a measure of acidity or alkalinity.

'PHAGE TYPING

See bacteriophage typing.

PLASMA

The colourless fluid part of the blood in which the cells are suspended.

PLATELETS

Cell fragments involved in blood clotting.

POLYMERASE CHAIN REACTION (PCR)
A technique which enables multiple copies of a DNA fragment to be generated by amplification of target DNA sequence.

PREVALENCE
The proportion of a population having a specific disease at a given point in time.

PRODROMAL
Relating to the period of time following the incubation period when the first symptoms of illness appear.

SELECTIVE MEDIA
Types of culture media which use selective agents such as antibiotics to inhibit some types of bacteria to allow the growth of others.

SEQUELAE
A condition which follows the occurrence of a disease e.g. late complications, permanent ill effects.

SERODIAGNOSIS
Identification of a micro-organism by means of serological tests.

SEROLOGY
The study of antigen-antibody reactions *in vitro*.

SEROTYPING
A method of distinguishing varieties of bacteria (serotypes) by defining their antigenic properties on the basis of their reaction to known antisera. A number of serotypes may constitute a serogroup.

SERUM ANTIBODIES
Antibodies found in the fluid fraction of coagulated blood.

SHIGA-LIKE TOXIN (SLT)
A term used synonymously with Verocytotoxin (VT) because VTs have an almost identical biological profile to the toxin produced by the "Shiga bacillus" (*Shigella dysenteriae*).

SOMATIC ANTIGEN
The antigen on the cell wall known as the "O" antigen.

SORBITOL MACCONKEY AGAR
A selective and differential medium for the detection of *Escherichia coli* O157:H7.

SPECIES
A classification of organisms within a genus which have similarities and can be further sub-divided into sub-species.

SPORADIC CASE
A single case of disease apparently unrelated to other cases.

STRAIN

A population of organisms within a species or sub-species distinguished by sub-typing.

SUB-SPECIES

A classification of organisms within a species which have similarities.

SUB-TYPING

Any method used to distinguish between species or sub-species.

SUSCEPTIBLE INDIVIDUAL

An individual who has no pre-existing immunity or resistance to infection who is therefore liable to become infected.

THROMBOTIC THROMBOCYTOPAENIA PURPURA (TTP)

A clinical condition resulting from the aggregation of platelets in various organs, and is characterised by fever with skin and central nervous involvement, anaemia and kidney failure.

TOXIN

Any poisonous substance produced by a micro-organism.

TYPING

Any method used to distinguish between closely related micro-organisms.

VEROCYTOTOXIN PRODUCING *ESCHERICHIA COLI* (VTEC)

A particular sub-species of *E.coli* often of the serogroup O157 which is associated with haemorrhagic colitis and haemolytic uraemic syndrome.

VIRULENCE

Virulence is defined broadly in terms of the severity of the symptoms in the host. Thus a highly virulent strain may cause severe symptoms in a susceptible individual, while a less virulent strain would produce relatively less severe symptoms in the same individual.

WATER ACTIVITY A_w

A measure of the available water in a substance.

Z-VALUE

The temperature coefficient of thermal destruction. It is the change in temperature (°C) which alters the D-value by a factor of 10.

APPENDIX 1

ADVISORY COMMITTEE ON THE MICROBIOLOGICAL SAFETY OF FOOD

LIST OF MEMBERS

CHAIRMAN

Professor Heather M Dick Professor of Medical Microbiology, University of Dundee

MEMBERS

Mr D Boon Director of Environmental Health and Trading Standards, London Borough of Croydon

Mr D Clarke Director of Quality Assurance, Purchasing and Supply, Forte plc

Professor R Feldman Professor of Clinical Epidemiology, London Hospital Medical College

Professor D L Georgala Independent Scientific Consultant; Retired Director of the Institute of Food Research

Dr R Gilbert Director of Food Hygiene Laboratory and Deputy Director of Central Public Health Laboratory, Public Health Laboratory Service

Dr P A Mullen Veterinary Adviser to Western United Investment Company

Dr M J Painter Consultant in Communicable Disease Control, City of Manchester

Professor S R Palmer Regional Consultant Epidemiologist, Communicable Disease Surveillance Centre, Welsh Unit, Cardiff Royal Infirmary

Ms B Saunders Consumer Consultant

Dr N Simmons Emeritus Consultant in Microbiology to the Guy's and St Thomas' Hospital Trust; Honorary Senior Lecturer in Microbiology, the London Hospital Medical College

Mr R Southgate Technical Executive, Northern Foods plc

Dr G Spriegel Director of Scientific Services, J Sainsbury plc

Dr M Stringer	Director of Food Science Division, Campden and Chorleywood Food Research Association
Dame Rachel Waterhouse	Formerly Chairman of Consumers' Association
Dr T Wilson	Senior Consultant Bacteriologist, Northern Ireland Public Health Laboratory, Belfast City Hospital

ASSESSORS

Mr B Bridges	Department of Health
Dr R J Cawthorne	Ministry of Agriculture, Fisheries and Food
Dr W H B Denner	Ministry of Agriculture, Fisheries and Food
Mr A J Matheson	Scottish Office Agriculture and Fisheries Department
Dr P Madden	Scottish Office Home and Health Department
Dr C H McMurray	Department of Agriculture for Northern Ireland
Dr E Mitchell	Department of Health and Social Services, Northern Ireland
Mr D Worthington	Welsh Office

SECRETARIAT

Dr C Swinson (Medical Secretary) (a)	Department of Health
Dr A Wight (Medical Secretary) (b)	Department of Health
Mr C R Mylchreest (Administrative Secretary)	Ministry of Agriculture, Fisheries and Food
Mr G M Robb (Minutes Secretary)	Department of Health

(a) Until June 1994
(b) From July 1994

APPENDIX 2

PATHOGENICITY DETERMINANTS

The pathogenicity of Verocytotoxin-producing strains of *E. coli* (VTEC) seems to be multifactorial and our current understanding suggests that at least two distinct mechanisms contribute to the pathogenesis of their disease manifestations. First, and by definition, they produce Verocytotoxins,[9, 17, 161, 162] and secondly, experiments in animals have shown that they possess a characteristic mechanism of attachment to intestinal cells that results in effacement (destruction) of microvilli.[27, 28, 161, 163] In addition, many strains elaborate an enterohaemolysin.[164]

Production of Verocytotoxins

A.2.1 Characteristic of all VTEC strains, regardless of serotype, is their ability to elaborate powerful cytotoxins, small (picogram) amounts of which cause irreversible damage to a variety of cell lines grown in tissue-culture. Vero (African Green Monkey kidney) cells have traditionally been used to demonstrate the presence of these cytotoxins which, therefore, are often called Verocytotoxins (VTs).[9, 17, 162, 165]

A.2.2 Most VTEC strains produce either, or both, of two principal Verocytotoxins, VT1 and VT2. In its physical, biological and antigenic properties, VT1 is almost identical to the Shiga toxin produced by strains of *Shigella dysenteriae* serotype 1 [19](the classical agent of bacillary dysentery); indeed, antiserum prepared against Shiga toxin (anti-Shiga-toxin) completely neutralises the activity of VT1. VT2, however, is antigenically distinct from VT1 and Shiga toxin and is not neutralised by anti-Shiga-toxin.[20, 166] The ability of some strains of *E. coli* to produce VT1 and VT2 is determined by genetic material carried on bacteriophages which may be transmitted to other strains along with the ability to elaborate VT1 and VT2.[20] Some VTEC strains from animals and man produce variant forms of VT2, most but not all, of which are neutralised by anti-VT2-serum and are not mediated by bacteriophages.[164, 167, 168]

A.2.3 The cytotoxicity of Shiga toxin, VT1 and VT2, readily detectable by their effects on Vero (and other) cells in tissue culture, may be demonstrated in other ways. When injected into ligated loops of the rabbit ileum, they cause fluid accumulation, i.e. are enterotoxic; and when injected into the peritoneum of mice, they cause paralysis of the hind legs and eventually death, i.e. are neurotoxic and lethal.[169]

A.2.4 These toxins are composed of A (active) and B (binding) subunits;[170] the latter mediate toxin binding by recognition of specific receptors present at the surface of susceptible cells. The receptor for most VTs is a glycolipid globotriaosyl ceramide (Gb$_3$);[171, 172, 173] some of the variant VT2s, however, bind better to globotetraosyl ceramide (Gb$_4$) than to Gb$_3$.[167, 168] Once attached to the surface receptor, the A subunit of the toxin enters the cell and inhibits protein synthesis, so that the target cells are eventually killed. It does this in a very specific way that is common to all VTs; cleavage of the glycosidic bond at site 4234 in the 28S ribosomal RNA of the 60S ribosomal subunit of host cells blocks elongation factor-1-dependent binding of aminoacyl-tRNA.[173, 174, 175, 176, 177]

A.2.5   VTs are likely to be important virulence determinants in several aspects of VTEC infection. For example, large amounts of VT can be detected in the faeces of patients with haemorrhagic colitis (HC) or haemolytic uraemic syndrome (HUS).[21] Killing of colonic epithelial cells by VT may contribute directly to fluid secretion and diarrhoea (but see below) and also, by damaging the blood vessels of the colon, cause the bloody diarrhoea characteristic of these conditions.

A.2.6   In most patients with HUS, damage is concentrated in the endothelium of the kidney; and in patients with more severe HUS, there is extensive damage to endothelial cells in other organs, e.g. the pancreas and the brain. Hence, endothelial cells are deemed to play an important role as major target cells in the pathogenesis of HC and HUS.[10, 18] Evidence of the susceptibility of endothelial cells comes from *in vitro* experiments with cultured, human umbilical vein endothelial cells (HUVEC) which are killed by the addition of VTs; killing is neutralised by anti-Shiga-toxin.[25]

A.2.7   Although VTs contribute to the development of HUS, additional stimuli are needed. Thus, it has been shown that HUVEC cells cultured *in vitro* are 10-100 times more sensitive to the action of VTs in the presence of inflammatory mediators, such as the lipopolysaccharide (LPS) endotoxin of the bacterial cell wall or cytokines, such as tumour necrosis factors (TNF) or interleukins [26] (e.g. IL-1). These inflammatory mediators are believed to stimulate the synthesis of more Gb_3 receptors at the endothelial cell surface, thereby increasing the amount of VT bound to target cells.[162] In this way, VTs and inflammatory mediators acting together cause more damage to endothelial cells than either does alone.[178]

A.2.8   Although the well-established association of VTEC with HUS suggests that circulating VT might play a major role in causing damage to kidneys and other tissues, convincing evidence for the presence of VT in the blood of patients with systemic VTEC infections is lacking. Even indirect evidence of systemic toxaemia, e.g. the development of antibodies to VTs in the serum of patients with HC or HUS, is controversial.[24, 179, 180]

A.2.9   It has been suggested that a B lymphocyte marker (CD77) has a similar structure to the receptor molecule for VT1 and VT2. This results in a binding of VT to B lymphocytes in lymphoid tissue which inhibits the antibody response to VT1 and VT2 and enables evasion of host antibody response.[181]

A.2.10   Nevertheless, evidence of circulating VT comes from experiments with rabbits injected intravenously with purified VT. Highly sensitive detection methods, such as radiolabelling and immunofluorescence, revealed localisation of toxin in the intestine, spinal cord and brain of the animals which also developed symptoms suggestive of involvement of the central nervous system. Some rabbits developed diarrhoea, consistent with the appearance of oedematous lesions in the caecum

96

together with some mucosal haemorrhaging, but the diarrhoea was not usually bloody.[22] Again, and in contrast with the histopathology of the kidneys of HUS patients that shows profound alterations of the glomeruli, the kidneys of the rabbits appeared normal and kidney functions were little, if at all, affected.[22] Thus, although this animal model provides evidence of circulating VT, it does not reproduce all the manifestations of the disease in man; rabbit kidneys probably lack receptors for toxin binding.[10]

A.2.11   In patients with HC, VTEC strains producing VT2 (alone or with VT1) may be more likely to develop the serious complications of HUS and TPP.[9, 182, 183] Is VT2, therefore, a relatively more important virulence determinant than VT1? Experiments with mice, injected intravenously or intraperitoneally with purified toxins, showed that VT2 was 400 times more lethal for mice than VT1; VT1, however, had greater affinity for Gb_3 (and Gb_4) receptors than VT2.[184] These studies suggested that the less active VT1 might bind preferentially to host tissues, such as colonic epithelial cells, low in Gb_3, thereby confining damage to the colonic epithelium and vasculature of the colon with resultant production of bloody diarrhoea. Blood-borne dissemination to distant sites might allow the more active VT2 toxin (even tiny amounts not detectable in blood) to damage tissues rich in Gb_3 receptors, e.g. the endothelial cells of the kidney, pancreas or brain.[184]

A.2.12   The receptor of VT1 and VT2 includes a terminal disaccharide (galactose-α-1→4-galactose) which, linked to ceramide or paragloboside, respectively, is also part of the blood-group antigens Pk and Pl.[185] Avid binding of VTs to red cells of these blood-group types might reduce the overall burden of VT available for uptake by the principal target cells, i.e. vascular endothelium, and explain why free VT is not detected in the blood of patients. There is some evidence from clinical observations that expression of Pl was reduced in children recovering from diarrhoea-associated HUS.[186]

Attachment and effacement mechanisms

A.2.13   Although lesions have been seen in colonic mucosa of man,[187] VTEC have not been found in human material obtained by biopsy or at necroscopy. Hence, very little is known about the colonisation of human intestinal tissues.[9] Moreover, in feeding experiments, VTEC of diverse serotypes colonised the terminal ileum, the caecum and the colon of experimental animals, such as rabbits and gnotobiotic piglets and calves.[188, 189]

A.2.14   VTEC also formed attaching and effacing (A/E) lesions in the intestines of these animals. Bacteria attached closely to the intestinal cell membranes which characteristically 'cupped' the bacteria to form structures known as 'pedestals'.[27, 28, 190, 191, 192] Within 3 days, effacement (destruction) of the microvillus border was seen, as much as 80% of the epithelial surface being damaged in some animals. Thereafter, deeper penetration by the bacteria through intercellular spaces resulted in ulceration and was accompanied by oedema in the deeper tissues. In these animal models, histological change was accompanied by symptoms of watery diarrhoea as the absorptive capacity of the microvilli was destroyed.[9, 30] The sequence of events is similar in natural infection of animals, e.g. in calves infected by a bovine strain of VTEC, except that in the latter case a bloody diarrhoea was produced.[9, 29] Similar A/E lesions have been seen in infections due to strains of enteropathogenic *E. coli* (EPEC), the classical agents of infantile diarrhoea.[193]

A.2.15   Attempts to unravel some aspects of the adhesion of VTEC to intestinal cells have been made with different cells grown in tissue-culture, with lines such as Hep2, CaCo2 and INT 407 of intestinal origin. These studies have suggested that attachment of VTEC to intestinal cells occurs in three stages.[194]

   i)   The initial attachment is mediated by a large plasmid (60 mDa in size) but it is unclear whether this loose attachment occurs via plasmid-encoded fimbriae or outer-membrane proteins (omp).[189, 195, 196]

   ii)   The more intimate binding that follows is determined by a chromosomal gene *eae* and is associated with the production of intimin, a 97 kDa omp showing much (83%) homology with the corresponding intimin of EPEC strains.[182] Intimin, though required, cannot itself produce the A/E lesions.[189, 195]

   iii) With the destruction of the microvilli immediately underlying the 'cupped' bacterium, a dense accumulation of host cytoskeletal elements, including filamentous actin, occurs giving rise to electron-dense adhesion pedestals.[193, 197] Additional, as yet unidentified, chromosomally determined gene products are required for this process which can be demonstrated by a positive fluorescent actin staining (FAS) reaction.[189, 195]

A.2.16   Some VTEC strains lack the ability to form A/E lesions. The adhesive mechanisms of these strains need to be assessed and their behaviour in tissue-culture and animal experiments needs to be evaluated.

Enterohaemolysin production

A.2.17   Many VTEC strains produce an enterohaemolysin thought to be correlated with possession of a large plasmid,[198] but the role of this putative determinant of virulence awaits definitive studies.

APPENDIX 3.1

LABORATORY DIAGNOSIS SURVEY

Introduction

A.3.1.1   In August 1993, 404 questionnaires were sent out by the VTEC Working Group to diagnostic/clinical laboratories in England and Wales. Laboratory addresses were chosen by selecting the name of the first microbiologist from each laboratory address in the Association of Medical Microbiologists Directory for 1992. In addition, 32 questionnaires were sent to NHS and university bacteriology laboratories in Scotland by CD(S)U (now SCIEH). Information was also collected from 14 clinical laboratories in N. Ireland by the Department of Health and Social Services (Northern Ireland). Following analysis of the response to the first posting, further questionnaires were sent out in January 1994 to laboratories which had not replied.

Results

A.3.1.2   Results from the survey are reported here and where appropriate comparisons are made with a previous survey covering England and Scotland reported by the PHLS in 1990.[32]

A.3.1.3   A total of 269 replies were received from England & Wales (225) Scotland (30) and N. Ireland (14). The response rate from England & Wales, excluding closed laboratories was 67%. The response rate for Scotland and N. Ireland was 100%, as all the questionnaires were followed up personally.

A.3.1.4   The replies were distributed between various types of laboratories (Table A.3.1).

Table A.3.1

Type of laboratory	No. replies
NHS, including NHS trust and Special Health Authorities	193
PHLS	53
Private	19
Military	3
University	1

A.3.1.5   Seventeen laboratories did not test for *E. coli* O157, but 10 of these referred specimens to other laboratories.

A.3.1.6   Two hundred and fifty-two (94%) laboratories in England, Wales, Scotland and Northern Ireland replied that they examined stool specimens for *E. coli* O157 which compares with 95% of laboratories in England and Scotland in the previous survey. Two hundred and thirteen (85%) laboratories selected stool samples for *E. coli* O157 testing by clinical or epidemiological criteria. Thirty-nine examined all stool samples (Table A.3.2).

Table A.3.2

	England & Wales	Scotland	N.Ireland	Total
Examine all samples	30	7	2	39
Select for examination	177	23	13	213

A.3.1.7   The criteria which laboratories applied for selection of samples to examine for *E. coli* O157 were bloody diarrhoea (85%), HUS (69%), colitis (13%), age < 16 years (14%), history of recent travel abroad (7%) and consumption of meat or beefburgers (2%). Most laboratories based their selection on bloody diarrhoea and HUS. Many laboratories also included a third criteria in the list as well as bloody diarrhoea and HUS. Similarly, the 1990 survey also found that the most common criteria for selection of samples were bloody diarrhoea and HUS.

A.3.1.8   Also, in common with the 1990 survey, the predominant isolation medium used was sorbitol MacConkey agar (SMAC) and most laboratories used O157 antiserum to identify suspect colonies. Five (2%) laboratories used cefixime rhamnose SMAC (CR-SMAC), 15 (6%) laboratories tested for Verocytotoxin and 7 (3%) used a DNA probe for the detection of VT genes.

A.3.1.9   The isolation rate from laboratories selecting for testing ranged from 0.04% to 1.3% giving a mean of 0.4%. The isolation rate from laboratories testing all samples ranged from 0.02% to 0.23% giving a mean of 0.1%. Several laboratories were unable to report the total number of samples they tested for *E. coli* O157 in 1992, these have been excluded from the annexes and calculations of isolation rates.

A.3.1.10   In 1992, 227 (90%) of the responding laboratories reported isolates to CDSC or CD(S)U, this was comparable to the percentage reporting in 1990.

A.3.1.11   In 1992, 218 (87%) referred clinical isolates to PHLS' Laboratory of Enteric Pathogens (LEP) or Aberdeen Royal Infirmary for confirmation and further typing. This is similar to the percentage who referred to PHLS' Division of Enteric Pathogens (DEP), now LEP, in 1990 (90%). The Scottish reference laboratory for VTEC was established in 1993.

A.3.1.12   In Table A.3.3, isolation rates for 1992 are given for Scotland, Wales, Northern Ireland and for each Regional Health Authority area in England, together with the comparable isolation rates for 1989 found in the previous survey.[32]

Region	Isolation[1] rate **with** selection		Isolation[1] rate **without** selection		Combined isolation[1] rate for 1992	Combined isolation[1] rate for 1989
Northern	39/7599,	**0.51%**	3/5830,	**0.05%**	0.3%	1.2%
North Western	43/20246,	**0.21%**	17/14000,	**0.12%**	0.18%	0.1%
West Midlands	27/7718,	**0.35%**	4/5999,	**0.07%**	0.23%	0.4%
Yorkshire	35/26160,	**0.13%**	-		0.13%	1.5%
Mersey	15/3309,	**0.45%**	2/9000,	**0.02%**	0.14%	0.3%
Trent	73/7133,	**1.02%**	-		1.02%	1.5%
East Anglia	27/2092,	**1.29%**	-		1.30%	1.0%
Oxford	21/1740,	**1.21%**	-		1.21%	4.6%
N E Thames	10/1764,	**0.57%**	0/1000		0.36%	0%
N W Thames	6/1882,	**0.32%**	15/6476,	**0.23%**	0.25%	0.1%
S E Thames	19/2034,	**0.93%**	2/4000,	**0.05%**	0.35%	0.1%
S W Thames	18/6816,	**0.26%**	-		0.26%	0.3%
Wessex	20/11525,	**0.17%**	7/4054,	**0.17%**	0.17%	0.5%
South Western	28/10967,	**0.25%**	-		0.26%	0.5%
Scotland	95/11602,	**0.82%**	19/11723,	**0.16%**	0.49%	1.1%
Wales	2/4700,	**0.04%**	29/40676,	**0.07%**	0.07%	-
N Ireland	4/2350,	**0.17%**	0/800		0.13%	-

[1] = Isolation rates are quoted for the number of samples positive for *E. coli* O157, using the total number of stool samples examined for *E. coli* O157 as the denominator.

A.3.1.13 Thirty-eight laboratories (15%) had changed their selection criteria since April 1991. Only 20 laboratories ((8%) reported carrying out more tests for *E. coli* O157 since April 1991.

A.3.1.14 Eighty-eight (35%) of the responding laboratories also tested foods, 89 (35%) tested milks and 72 (29%) tested waters. Of those testing food, 44 (17%) laboratories reported that they tested selected foods for *E. coli* O157, while only 3 (1%) tested all food samples for *E. coli* O157.

A.3.1.15 Reference laboratories were requested most commonly to 'phage type isolates, test for VT production and VT genes.

A.3.1.16 One hundred and eighty-seven (94%) laboratories did not carry out tests for O157 antibodies.

Summary and Conclusions

A.3.1.17 Approximately the same percentage of laboratories examined stool samples for *E. coli* O157 in 1992 as in 1989. Some had changed their selection criteria and some examined all specimens.

A.3.1.18 The spread of geographical variation in isolation rates for 1992 is less than that found in 1989, 0.07% to 1.3% in 1992 compared with 0% to 4.6% in 1989. Ten out of 14 RHAs in England and Scotland reported lower isolation rates in 1992 compared to 1989.

A.3.1.19 Oxford still had a high isolation rate (1.2%) compared to other regions but not as high as that reported in 1989 (4.6%). Those regions that had changed markedly were; Northern with a decrease from 1.2% to 0.3% and Yorkshire with a decrease from 1.5% to 0.13%. The isolation rate in Scotland had decreased from 1.1% to 0.49%. Wales and Northern Ireland were not included in the 1989 survey but both had low rates of isolation for 1992.

A.3.1.20 The overall combined isolation rate found in this survey for the UK for 1992 was 0.4%, this is lower than in the 1989 survey which was 0.7%. The calculation of the isolation rate for the 1989 survey was based on replies from 130 laboratories and a stool sample denominator of 29,487, giving a mean of 227 tests per laboratory. The calculation of the isolation rate for the 1992 survey was based on replies from 252 laboratories and a stool sample denominator figure of 238,708, giving a mean of 947 tests per laboratory. Although the 1992 isolation rate from the stool samples that were tested has gone down compared to 1989, the actual number of isolates of *E. coli* O157 has increased because more stool samples were tested.

A.3.1.21 As stool denominator figures are only available through laboratory diagnosis questionnaires, isolation rates which are estimations of infection rates, are often made using the number of laboratory reports of a particular pathogen per 100,000 head of population. Calculated in this way the isolation rate per 100,000 head of population in England and Wales was 0.23 in 1989 and 0.92 in 1992.[33] The results of this questionnaire indicate that it is possible that an increase in ascertainment i.e. more stool samples tested for *E. coli* O157 could have caused this apparent increase in isolation rate.

APPENDIX 3.2

AD HOC PAEDIATRIC HUS SURVEY IN THE UK

Introduction

A.3.2.1   Fifty-five letters were sent to members of the British Association of Paediatric Nephrology (see 3.26) on behalf of the Working Group requesting:

1) figures from clinical practice on the number of cases of HUS seen by units over the last decade; and

2) any information on the cause and outcome of these cases.

Results

A.3.2.2   Out of the 24 units represented, 21 replies were received giving a response rate of 87%. Nine replies did not provide any figures. Out of these 9, one was excluded because it came from outside the UK (Eire).

A.3.2.3   Twelve replies provided information in variable detail which is listed as follows:

Birmingham (referral centre)
-          1-16 cases per annum HUS (125 in 14 years).
           O157 data available since 1985. 7 deaths recorded.

Bristol (referral centre)
-          1-9 cases per annum HUS (46 in 7 1/2 years). (No obvious trend).

Cardiff (referral centre)
-          3-4   cases per annum HUS (range 0-10 years). VTEC established in approximately 1/3 of cases.

Great Ormond Street Hospital for Sick Children, London (referral centre)
-          < 10 cases per annum (1966-1984)
-          12-16 cases per annum (1985-1992)
-          VTEC established in 16 out of 69 cases between 1985-1992.
-          D+ HUS (188 in 26 years)

Guy's Hospital, London. (referral centre)
-          2-16 cases per annum HUS (97 in 10 years).
           VTEC established in 19 cases (9/15 in 1992). 2 deaths recorded.

Kettering
-          1-2 cases per annum HUS

Nottingham (referral centre)
-         8-14 cases per annum HUS (87 in 8 years).

Oxford
-         1 case per annum, outcomes good.

Portsmouth
-         1-2 cases per annum HUS (14 in 10 years).
         O157 established in 3 cases.

Royal Free Hospital, London
-         1989 - 1 case
         1990 - 1 case
         1991 - 7 cases
         1992 - 8 cases

St Mary's Hospital Medical School
-         no cases in last 2-3 years.
-         any cases prior to this would have been referred to Great Ormond Street and Guy's Hospitals.

Sheffield
-         1993 only } - 5 cases HUS - 4 VTEC
                   - 2 VTEC infections, no HUS.

Conclusions

A.3.2.4   It is difficult to draw any firm conclusions about a change in the incidence of HUS, particularly in relation to VTEC infection, for the following reasons:

- the data is incomplete both nationally and also within individual centres;

- there are no consistent time periods to compare;

- in most cases no information is available on cause;

- it is not possible to determine a trend from these limited data.

These findings confirm the value of a national prospective surveillance study with clearly defined aims. However, contrary to the expectations of the Working Group, there is no firm evidence over the last ten years of an increase in the number of cases of HUS.

104

LARGE OUTBREAK IN THE WESTERN USA IN 1992-1993 AND SUBSEQUENT CONTROL MEASURES

Introduction

A.3.3.1   In January 1993 a large outbreak of *E. coli* O157 was identified in Washington State. Clinicians at the Children's Hospital and Medical Centre, Seattle became alerted to an increase in the number of visits to the emergency room by children with bloody diarrhoea as well as an increase in the number of HUS patients being referred from local hospitals. Smaller outbreaks in Nevada, California, and Idaho were subsequently identified and the same vehicle, hamburgers consumed at multiple outlets of a single restaurant chain, were thought to be responsible. A total of 732 patients were affected, and of these, 195 were hospitalised and 55 developed HUS or TTP. There were 4 deaths. In Washington State, 614 patients were involved of whom 491 were culture positive. The stools of the remaining 123 patients with HC and/or HUS were either negative (75) or not tested (48). Fifty-eight cases (11.8%) were determined to be secondary to cases who contracted the disease via consumption of a contaminated hamburger. The median age of patients was 7.5 years (range 0-74); 35 patients developed HUS and 3 died.[75, 76, 199]

Laboratory diagnosis of human *E. coli* O157:H7 infection

A.3.3.2   Almost all patients who reported for medical attention with enteric symptoms were asked to submit stool samples for bacterial culture. Culture was not limited to patients with bloody diarrhoea. However, the vast majority of patients whose culture did yield *E. coli* O157:H7 did have gross blood in their stool (personal communication from Dr Tarr, Washington State). One child excreted the organism for 72 days and may have been an asymptomatic carrier. Anti-LPS (*E. coli* O157) was detected in 95% of available unpaired serum samples. Anti-VT response was detected in 20% of samples using an ELISA plus toxin neutralisation test.

A.3.3.3   In order to determine if the *E. coli* O157:H7 human outbreak isolates were the same strain or a mixture of strains a variety of techniques were used. Centers for Disease Control and Prevention (CDC) looked at 70 human samples and found that the outbreak strain was Lior's 'phage type 14 and produced both Verocytotoxin 1 and 2. Plasmid profiling was done but was deemed not to be discriminatory enough from previous experience. Pulsed field gel electrophoresis (PFGE) using both *Xba* I and *Avr* II enzymes was known to give good discrimination from previous work and results using this method agreed with other sub-typing methods that all but two clinical isolates were the same strain.

A.3.3.4   Washington State used a new sub-typing technique.[200] This technique involved extracting total DNA from the isolate and performing restriction fragment length polymorphism (RFLP) analysis using the enzyme *Pvu* II. After RFLP analysis, the gels were probed with a lambda 'phage probe. The technique had been previously used on 47 *E. coli* O157:H7 isolates collected from sporadic cases of HUS and HC and gave 39 unique profiles. Using the same technique with 400 outbreak isolates, 395 isolates gave identical profiles.

E. coli O157:H7 isolation from implicated food

A.3.3.5   Implicated lots of minced beef were confiscated by State and County Public Health Authorities. These food samples were tested by Professor M P Doyle of the University of Georgia, Washington State and US Department of Agriculture (USDA). Even though different methods were used, many of the samples were tested by all the laboratories and the sensitivity of detection was found to be comparable.

A.3.3.6   The method used by Professor Doyle involved enrichment of 25g of food in selective enrichment medium for 18 hours at 37°C with agitation. The enrichment culture was then used in an ELISA with a polyclonal capture antibody specific for *E. coli* O157 antigen and a monoclonal antibody specific for serotypes O157:H7 and O26:H11 as detection antibody.[124] This ELISA, which is the basis of the Organon Teknika EHEC-TEK kit, was first used to identify the *E. coli* O157:H7 positive minced beef samples and then all colonies typical of *E. coli* O157:H7 on sorbitol MacConkey agar plates with MUG were identified biochemically and serologically.

A.3.3.7   Washington State's isolation technique used a protocol based on standard microbiological techniques analysing sorbitol non-fermenting colonies and lactose fermenting colonies isolated from the minced beef samples. Candidate colonies were then further analysed for their indole positivity and possession of VT1 and VT2 genes. Isolates recovered from the incriminated meat and from 61 (96.8%) of 63 patients possessed the same lambda 'phage RFLP profile.[200] It was estimated that the incriminated patties contained on average, only approximately several hundred *E. coli* O157:H7. It was also estimated that 1 in 300-400 patties served produced clinically apparent infection (personal communication Dr P Tarr).

A.3.3.8   The standard method used by the USDA was the 3M Petrifilm™ for presumptive testing.[201] The method involves the inoculation of sample into an enrichment broth, incubation for 8 hours at 37°C with agitation followed by inoculation of 3M Petrifilm™ *E. coli* count plates, then identification by biochemical and serological tests of suspect colonies. Other methods used were the dipstick ELISA,[202] conventional direct culture onto SMAC and use of different enrichment broths. Other tests used to establish the general sanitary condition of the meat were total viable counts, total coliform counts, aerobic plate counts and detection of *Staphylococcus aureus*.

A.3.3.9   Most probable number analyses of *E. coli* O157:H7 on meat samples indicated 1-15 organisms/g. If the average hamburger is 40g this would give an infectious dose of 40-600 organisms per uncooked hamburger suggesting that the infectious dose was low in a cooked hamburger.[14, 203] There was no evidence that the outbreak strain was particularly pathogenic and it seems likely that host characteristics accounted for the spectrum of human disease seen in the outbreak.

A.3.3.10   The predominant view held by the Washington State epidemiologists and USDA and FDA officials, was that the only Verocytotoxin producing *E. coli* of importance to human disease was O157:H7. This is contrary to the view held in Canada and the UK. In the US it is accepted that other Verocytotoxin producing *E. coli* other than O157:H7 can cause human disease. However, present detection technology poses many obstacles to efficient and economical diagnosis of non-O157 serogroups and efforts needed to be concentrated solely on O157.

Occurrence of *E. coli* O157 in cattle

A.3.3.11   In October 1992 the USDA Food Safety Inspection Service started the Nationwide Beef Microbiological Baseline Data Collection Program.[204] The objectives of this programme are:

- to collect data for developing and maintaining a general, ongoing microbiological description or "profile" of fed cattle (steer and heifer) carcases for a number of micro-organisms (including *E. coli* O157:H7) of public concern and;

- to use the information and knowledge gained from this programme as a reference for further investigations and evaluation of new prevention programmes.

As USDA expect the prevalence in carcases to be about 0.1% it is unlikely that routine testing will be justifiable and more value was to be gained from assessing the prevalence of *E. coli* O157:H7 infection in herds.

A.3.3.12   A bovine surveillance programme was conducted in Washington State during 1990 to 1992. This concentrated on *E. coli* O157 rather than all VTECs as human exposure to other VTECs in food is much more common than *E. coli* O157, yet most human disease is attributed to *E. coli* O157. The programme found *E. coli* O157:H7 in 10 of 3750 (0.28%) faecal samples from 5 out of 60 dairy herds (8.3%) and from 10 of 1412 (0.7%) faecal samples from beef cattle in 4 of 25 (16%) cow/calf herds. The same study identified certain cattle management practices, such as computerized feeders and irrigation of pastures with manure slurry that were associated with the occurrence of *E. coli* O157:H7 on dairy farms.[107, 108]

107

Investigation of the source of the outbreak

A.3.3.13   The Federal investigation of the outbreak was co-ordinated between CDC and USDA. USDA and CDC each carried out a meat traceback with the purpose of identifying specific animals from which the meat product was derived. Five traceback steps were identified:

- the processing plant that produced the *E. coli* O157:H7 culture positive hamburger patties;

- all sources of boneless meat used in the production of the patties;

- the slaughterhouses that produced the carcases from which the boneless meat was derived;

- the feedlots (US method of farming beef) and markets which supplied the livestock to the slaughterhouses; and

- the farms where the livestock were raised.

A.3.3.14   The most often identified food source among those who became ill during the outbreak was hamburger patties sold by a single restaurant chain. The hamburger processing plant was quickly identified because it was the only producer of the restaurant chain's hamburgers. The Washington Public Health Authorities epidemiologically identified the product produced at the hamburger processing plant on 19 November 1992 as the vehicle of the pathogen. All returned product was made available for microbiological testing to a number of laboratories participating in the investigation. Results of the microbiological testing agreed with the epidemiological findings as most of the contaminated meat was found to be processed on 19 November for regular size patties. The rest of the contaminated meat was processed on 20 November for jumbo size patties.

A.3.3.15   Meat samples and equipment swabs were taken from approximately 20 slaughter and processing plants known to have been suppliers to the hamburger processing plant. It was possible to trace the source of the contaminated meat to a number of abattoirs' cutting plants but USDA could not determine more specifically the origin of the contaminated meat. Part of the problem lay in the imprecise documentation supplied by the processing plant concerning the batch formulation (product in) of finished product lots (product out). This meant that USDA and CDC were unable to identify the supplier source of the contaminated meat and therefore unable to traceback to any specific farm, herd or animal.[14]

A.3.3.16   No samples were taken in the restaurant, although in Nevada, simulated cooking procedures showed that the correct temperatures were not being reached. Cooked hamburgers inspected by sanitarians in Washington State were pink and when probed for temperature were below 68.3°C (155°F).

Control and prevention measures

United States Department of Agriculture (USDA)

A.3.3.17   A recall of all the product distributed from the restaurant chain's warehouses was initiated on 18 January. More than 100,000 lbs of hamburger patties were confiscated by USDA. As there was no effective way of testing all potentially contaminated meat to ensure safety it would either be destroyed or reworked into an animal feed product. The USDA report of the outbreak, May 1993, states that "insanitary slaughter and dressing procedures led to the contamination".[14]

A.3.3.18   There was a suggestion during the meat traceback exercise that some of the smaller slaughterhouses supplying meat to the processing plant used methods which may have contributed to the contamination of carcases with *E. coli* O157:H7. These included the use of bed slaughter, meat handling practices that could result in faecal contamination e.g. infrequent sterilisation of knives and saws. As a result, USDA expanded its review of slaughter houses via its Progressive Enforcement Action (PEA) programme which can withdraw federal inspection and close plants if plants are identified as having deficiencies in hygienic practice.

A.3.3.19   USDA accelerated the implementation of the Food Safety Inspection Service Pathogen Reduction Programme (PRP).[205] This programme aims to reduce the likelihood that harmful micro-organisms such as *Salmonella, Listeria monocytogenes* or *E. coli* O157:H7 will enter the food supply at key points in the production, distribution and consumption chain. The plan that USDA is adopting is based on HACCP principles and incorporates the essential elements of a pathogen reduction approach. This includes critical "pre-harvest" production activities, research on rapid methods which can be used in meat processing plants, "post-harvest" research in slaughter and processing plants, food service and retail activities and aggressive consumer education.

A.3.3.20   As part of the Pathogen Reduction Program, the USDA is seeking legislative changes to mandate animal identification and traceback to enhance future epidemiological investigations. The USDA FSIS amended the Federal meat and poultry products inspection regulations by mandating the inclusion of safe handling instructions (see page 110) on the labels of all imported and domestic raw meat and poultry to indicate the microbiological hazards associated with handling raw meat.[206, 207] The use of trisodium phosphate, chlorine or organic acid sanitation processes for beef carcases and irradiation and pasteurisation of fresh minced beef is being investigated.

SAFE HANDLING INSTRUCTIONS

"This product was inspected for your safety. Some animal products may contain bacteria that could cause illness if the product is mishandled or cooked improperly. For your protection, follow these safe handling instructions.

- **Keep refrigerated or frozen.**
  Thaw in refrigerator or microwave.

- **Keep raw meats or poultry separate from other foods. Wash working surfaces (including cutting boards), utensils and hands after touching raw meat or poultry.**

- **Cook thoroughly.**

- **Refrigerate left-overs within 2 hours."**

Food and Drug Administration (FDA)

A.3.3.21   The FDA is responsible for control and inspection at the retail end of the food chain. Although the FDA issues guidance to the states it is up to the individual states to incorporate it into legislation.

A.3.3.22   In November 1992 FDA recommended in the Model Food Code Provisions "that the temperature of potentially hazardous foods should be less than 7°C or more than 60°C at all times". During the outbreak, interim advice was given that minced beef products should be cooked to heat all parts of the food to 68.3°C (155°F), and this has been incorporated into the Food Code 1993.[140, 157, 158, 206]

A.3.3.23   Most restaurants do a test run in the morning by cooking hamburgers and testing the temperature with probes. The calibration of the grill can then be adjusted if necessary. This would be a CCP under a HACCP system. It would be up to the restaurant chains to give their outlets instructions about cooking and temperature control. State investigators and federal investigators can verify temperatures and any records kept if they inspect restaurants.

Centers for Disease Control and Prevention (CDC)/National Center for Infectious Disease (NCID)

A.3.3.24   Since the outbreak CDC/NICD have published a leaflet entitled "Preventing Foodborne Illness: *E. coli* O157:H7" with the purpose of educating the public at large about the organism, its spread, types of illness it causes, how illness is diagnosed and treated, the long-term consequences of infection and prevention of infection.[208] Under the heading "What can you do to prevent *E. coli* O157:H7 infection?" five points are made which are listed as follows:

-   Cook all minced beef or hamburger thoroughly. Make sure that the cooked meat is grey or brown throughout (not pink), any juices run clear, and the inside is hot;

-   If you are served an undercooked hamburger in a restaurant, send it back and ask for further cooking;

-   Consume only pasteurised milk and milk products. Avoid raw milk;

-   Make sure that infected persons, especially children, wash their hands carefully and frequently with soap to reduce the risk of spreading the infection; and

-   Drink municipal water that had been treated with adequate levels of chlorine or other effective disinfectants.

US industry perspective and public awareness after the outbreak

A.3.3.25   As a result of the outbreak some producers wanted research done into preventive measures, others did not accept that cattle were proven reservoirs of the pathogen. Some restaurant chains required suppliers to provide meat tested free from *E. coli* O157. However, this meant that meat which was not tested free could still end up on retail sale in supermarkets. Some parts of the food industry were willing to implement control measures and had done so, e.g. some restaurant chains had now installed a standardised method (clamp shell) for the effective heat-treatment of their hamburgers. As public awareness of *E. coli* O157 grew, the industry feared that meat consumption would be adversely affected.

A.3.3.26   After the outbreak there was more public awareness of *E. coli* O157 and sporadic cases were being reported in the media. The public regarded hamburgers as potentially unsafe food and were shocked that the Government had not prevented meat from becoming contaminated with *E. coli* O157. The American public make a considerable amount of hamburgers at home using minced beef and there was, therefore, more concern about sporadic cases than outbreaks because potential outbreaks in fast food restaurants were controllable by the food industry. Public education about proper cooking and cross-contamination was deemed to be important.

APPENDIX 3.4

SURVEY OF SURVEILLANCE/RESEARCH IN SOME MEMBER STATES OF THE EUROPEAN UNION

Introduction

A.3.4.1   The Working Group sent out a request for information on surveillance and research on VTEC to 24 government institutions and research establishments in 11 EC countries. Eight replies were received 3 of which were nil returns. The following is a summary of the information supplied.

GERMANY

E. coli Reference Laboratory, Robert Koch-Institut des Bundesgesundheitsamtes (National Health Institute)

A.3.4.2   The reference laboratory was established in 1992. Currently there are no official notification regulations for human or animal infections due to *E. coli*. The reference laboratory receives putative VTEC strains for confirmation and characterization from collaborating diagnostic laboratories in Germany. The strains are characterised biochemically, serologically and for presence of virulence markers, Verocytotoxins, haemolysins and adherence properties. Most of the VTEC isolates received which originate from humans are serotypes O26:H11, O111:H8 and O157:H7.

A.3.4.3   Enterohaemolysin production was first described in the German *E. coli* Reference Laboratory and the laboratory is continuing to investigate enterohaemolysin as a virulence marker of enterohaemorrhagic and enteropathogenic *E. coli*.

A.3.4.4   The laboratory has investigated the prevalence of VTEC in faecal samples in 7 different species of healthy domestic animals (cattle, sheep, goats, chickens, dogs, cats and pigs). VTEC were isolated from 208 animals (28.9%) and were most frequent in samples from sheep (66.6%), goat (56.1%) and cattle (21.1%). VTEC occurred more sporadically in pigs (7.5%), cats (13.8%) and dogs (4.8%) and were not isolated at all from chickens. A total of 41 different O:H serotypes were isolated with 54.8% represented by serotypes O5:H-, O91:H-, O146:H21, O128:H2 and OX3:H8. Nearly 60% of all VTEC O:H serotypes isolated in the study have been implicated as human pathogens indicating that healthy domestic animals could serve as a reservoir of human VTEC pathogens. All VTEC isolates except 9 feline strains hybridised with VT1 and VT2 specific DNA probes. Verocytotoxin and enterohaemolysin production were associated in those *E. coli* isolated from goats, sheep and cattle. Only 30 of 240 (12.5%) enterohaemolysin producing strains hybridised with an enterohaemolysin specific DNA probe indicating a heterogeneity in regulatory or structural enterohaemolysin genes in the strains of *E. coli* examined (personal communication Dr L Beutin).

112

Institute for Meat Hygiene, Free University of Berlin

A.3.4.5   Several lines of research into VTEC are underway at the Institute. These include the assessment of different enrichment procedures, quantitative estimation of VTEC strains in foods using gene probes and the characterisation of VTEC strains using PCR techniques with different primers.

A.3.4.6   In a study investigating 423 food samples, 71% were found to be positive for *E. coli* but none were O157. Using a colony hybridisation technique and a gene probe specific for VT1 and VT2, only 3 VTEC strains were detected in 1809 isolates. The VTEC positive strains originated from 2 samples of minced beef and 1 sample of raw milk cheese. The detection rate of VTEC in all food samples tested was 0.7%; in food samples originating from cattle it was 1.8%.

A.3.4.7   At the end of the study the conclusion was that there was negligible danger to the German consumer as the rate of VTEC isolations from foods of animal origin was low (personal communication Dr M Bülte).

DENMARK

The Danish Veterinary Serum Laboratory - Danish Veterinary Service

A.3.4.8   The Danish serum laboratory has carried out a presumptive estimation of the prevalence of VTEC in clinical material from cattle and pigs. DNA techniques for the detection of Verocytotoxin genes VT1, VT2 and VT2v have also been developed.

A.3.4.9   In calves, 26 (8.4%) of the *E. coli* strains from clinical cases of diarrhoea were VT positive. In material from cattle sampled at slaughter, 19 (13%) out of 150 meat and faecal samples were VT positive with 3 of the positive samples being from meat. Some of the Verocytotoxin positive strains were serotyped and 2 of these strains were identified as O157:H7. In pigs, Verocytotoxin genes were detected in 18 (9.4%) of the *E. coli* strains from neonatal diarrhoea and 52 (21.7%) of the *E. coli* strains from weaning diarrhoea. The Danish group conclude that potential human pathogenic *E. coli* strains can be found in the animal reservoir in Denmark (personal communication Dr L Rasmussen).

NETHERLANDS

Inspectorate for Health Protection - Food Inspection Service

A.3.4.10   Research has focused on techniques for the detection and isolation of Verocytotoxin producing *E. coli* in retail meat samples. Methods used were enrichment in modified tryptone soya broth plus acriflavine followed by plating onto sorbitol MacConkey agar, the 3M Petrifilm™ technique and, a polymerase chain reaction (PCR) for Verocytotoxigenic *E. coli* .[209] *E. coli* O157 positive strains were isolated from 22 (6.1%) of 360 samples of meat and chicken products. All O157 positive samples were negative for Verocytotoxicity and lacked the H7 antigen.

A.3.4.11   The PCR assay was used to examine 180 beef samples for the presence of the Shiga-like toxins SLT 1 and SLT 2. A total of 29 (16%) showed a positive reaction. Serotyping of the VTEC strains isolated from enrichment cultures showed that none were O157:H7, but serotypes O8:K?, O22:K-, O71:K-, O75:K1, O88:K-, O101:K(A)?, O123:K? were represented. Overall, some 1200 raw meat samples have been examined by the research group but *E. coli* O157:H7 has not yet been isolated (personal communication Dr E de Boer).

SPAIN

Spanish Ministry for Health and Consumption

A.3.4.12   An Enterobacteriaceae reference laboratory is located in the National Centre for Health Microbiology, Virology and Immunology in the Carlos Institute of Health, Madrid. The analytical methods employed in Spanish laboratories for the detection of VTEC include serotyping, detection of cytotoxins using Vero and HeLa cells, immunoblotting and ELISA techniques (personal communication Dr M A Usera).

APPENDIX 4.1

METHODS FOR O157 VTEC

Isolation/detection methods for clinical samples

A.4.1.1   Most clinical laboratories test for O157 VTEC by plating faecal specimens on MacConkey agar plates containing 1% D-sorbitol instead of lactose as, unlike most *E. coli*, O157 VTEC do not ferment sorbitol within 24 hours.[210]   VTEC of serogroup O157 produce non-sorbitol fermenting colonies that are small, round, smooth and may look greyish.   Non-sorbitol fermenting colonies are tested for agglutination with an O157 antiserum or with an O157 latex agglutination kit.[211, 212, 213]

A.4.1.2   Modifications of the sorbitol MacConkey agar (SMAC) have been described with the aim of improving the selectivity for O157 VTEC.   In one medium cefixime and rhamnose were incorporated into SMAC agar.[214]   O157 VTEC do not ferment rhamnose on agar plates in 24 hours, whereas many non-sorbitol fermenting *E. coli* of other serogroups do ferment rhamnose; cefixime is included because it is active against *Proteus* spp. frequently found in faeces.   Other media contain fluorogenic or chromogenic glucuronides in the SMAC agar to allow detection of ß-glucuronidase production.[201, 215]   The vast majority of O157 VTEC do not produce ß-glucuronidase whereas most other *E. coli* are positive in this test.[216, 217] Recently, another modification has been described in which the SMAC agar contains tellurite and cefixime,[218] because minimum inhibitory concentrations (MICs) were higher for O157 VTEC than for other *E. coli* and for non-sorbitol fermenters such as *Aeromonas*, *Plesiomonas*, *Morganella* and *Providencia*. Details of the media are shown in Table A.4.1.

A.4.1.3   Reports from Germany have described O157 VTEC strains that ferment sorbitol in 24 hours and produce ß-glucuronidase.[219, 220]   Such strains have not been detected in the UK but would not have been identified using the methods described in A.4.1.1 and A.4.1.2

Isolation/detection methods for food samples

A.4.1.4   O157 VTEC are usually isolated directly from faeces but for food and environmental samples growth in liquid medium is usually employed to increase the number of target organisms.   Standard methods using 44°C for the selective isolation of *E. coli* from foods are unsatisfactory because O157 VTEC grow very poorly at 44°C.[128]   Several liquid media for the enrichment of O157 VTEC have been reported and some are listed in Table A.4.2.   Modified trypticase soy broth is supplemented with either novobiocin or acriflavin to reduce the growth of Gram-positive organisms.   Another enrichment medium is buffered peptone water with vancomycin, cefsulodin and cefixime to suppress the growth of Gram-positive organisms, *Aeromonas* spp. and *Proteus* spp. respectively.   Optimal recovery of O157 VTEC was obtained with growth for 6 hours.[212]

115

TABLE A.4.1

SOLID MEDIA

DESIGNATION	COMPOSITION	REFERENCE
SMAC	MacConkey agar D-sorbitol, 1%	Farmer and Davis [210]
CR-SMAC	MacConkey sorbitol agar (Oxoid) Rhamnose, 0.5% Cefixime, 0.05mg/litre	Chapman et al.[214]
CT-SMAC	MacConkey sorbitol agar (Oxoid) Cefixime, 0.05mg/litre Potassium tellurite, 2.5mg/litre	Zadik et al.[218]
MSA-MUG	MacConkey sorbitol agar (Difco) MUG, 0.01%	Padhye and Doyle [124]
PRS-MUG	Phenol red base + 2% agar D-sorbitol, 0.5% 4-methylumbelliferyl β-D-glucuronide, 0.005%	Okrend et al.[201, 221]
MSA-BC1G	MacConkey sorbitol agar (Difco) 5-bromo-4-chloro-3-indoxyl- β-D-glucuronic acid cyclohexylammonium salt, 0.01%	Okrend et al.[201, 215]
HC	Tryptone, 20g/litre Bile salts 3, 1.12g/litre Sodium chloride (NaCl) 5g/litre Sorbitol, 20g/litre MUG, 0.01% Bromocresol purple, 0.015g/litre	Szabo et al.[222]

TABLE A.4.2

LIQUID MEDIA

DESIGNATION	COMPOSITION (PER LITRE)	REFERENCE
mTSB	Trypticase soy broth, 30g Bile salts 3, 1.5g Dipotassium phosphate (K_2HPO_4), 1.5g Novobiocin, 20mg	Doyle and Schoeni [123]
dm TSB-CA*	Trypticase soy broth, 30g Bile salts 3, 1.5g K_2HPO_4 1.5g Casamino acids, 10g Acriflavin-HCl, 10mg	Padhye and Doyle [124]
BPW-VCC	Buffered peptone water (Oxoid) Vancomycin, 8mg Cefixime, 0.05mg Cefsulodin, 10mg	Chapman et al.[102]
mEC+n	Tryptone, 20g Bile salts 3, 1.12g Lactose, 5g K_2HPO_4, 4g KH_2PO_4, 1.5g NaCl, 5g Novobiocin, 20mg	Organon Teknika [223]

* This medium has been modified for testing dairy products by addition of Na_2HPO_4 (6g/litre) and KH_2PO_4 (1.35g/litre) instead of K_2HPO_4 (1.5g/litre).[223]

A.4.1.5 After growth in enrichment media a number of methods can be used to detect *E. coli* O157 strains. Immunomagnetic separation uses beads coated with polyclonal *E. coli* O157 antibodies.[212, 224] These beads are now commercially available (Dynal). After enrichment the beads are usually cultured on one of the media listed in Table A.4.1.

A.4.1.6 Colony immunoblotting has also been employed to detect *E. coli* O157.[119] After enrichment, cultures are spread on agar plates and colonies are transferred to nitrocellulose membranes. An alkaline phosphatase-conjugated O157 antiserum is used for the detection of positive colonies. A commercially available blot ELISA method (3M Corporation) has been developed for the detection of the O157 antigen. This test has been used for testing of foods by the United States Department of Agriculture.

A.4.1.7 A rapid sandwich enzyme-linked immunosorbent assay (ELISA) has been described for the detection of O157 VTEC in foods.[124] In this test polyclonal O157 antibody is used as the capture antibody and a monoclonal antibody, claimed to be specific for VTEC belonging to serogroups O157 and O26, is used as the detection antibody. The reagents are now available as a kit (Organon Teknika). Samples that are positive in this ELISA need to be examined further to isolate the putative O157 VTEC.

A.4.1.8 O157 VTEC can be detected directly from faecal specimens in less than 2 hours by direct immunofluorescence antibody staining.[225] Optimum results were obtained with specimens that were treated with 5% bleach.

Confirmatory tests for *E. coli* O157 identification

A.4.1.9 Colonies that appear to be *E.coli* O157 must be confirmed as *E. coli* using biochemical tests. These should exclude any non-*E.coli* that give false positive agglutination tests with the O157 antiserum. *Escherichia hermanii* is biochemically and serologically similar to *E. coli* O157 and cross reacts with polyclonal antisera to *E. coli* O157.[226] However *E. coli*, unlike *E. hermanii*, does not ferment cellobiose and does not grow in the presence of potassium cyanide. In addition, strains of *E. hermanii* ferment rhamnose and are sensitive to tellurite and therefore would not be detected on CR-SMAC or CT-SMAC.[212, 213]

A.4.1.10 Strains that appear to be *E. coli* O157 should be confirmed serologically with antisera against O and H antigens. O157 VTEC usually have the flagellar antigen H7 although some strains are non-motile. All confirmed *E. coli* O157 strains should be tested for production of VT or the presence of VT genes (see next section).

Methods for the detection of Verocytotoxin production and VT genes

A.4.1.11 Verocytotoxin is detected by its cytotoxic effect on Vero cells.[17] Faecal suspensions, culture filtrates or live cultures can be tested.[227, 228] Strains are grown in trypticase soy broth and culture filtrates are added to monolayers of Vero cells. Cells round up and become detached in the presence of VT. Final readings are usually made after incubation for 3 to 4 days when the cells are fixed and stained. As an alternative to testing individual colonies broth inoculated with sweeps can be examined. To increase the sensitivity of the test it is recommended that VT obtained after polymyxin release is detected.[229]

A.4.1.12 To confirm that cytotoxic effects on Vero cells are due to the presence of VT, neutralization tests using antisera against VT1 or VT2 should be performed.[230] The heat-lability of the toxin should be confirmed by showing that VT tests on samples heated at 100°C for 15 minutes are negative. Samples from faeces can also be tested on a cell line which is not sensitive to VT such as Y1 mouse adrenal tumour cells. A sample that kills Y1 cells to the same titre as Vero cells is considered negative for VT, but VT present at a lower titre would not be detected.

A.4.1.13 Several ELISAs have been described for the detection of VT.[231, 232, 233] Some bind VT to glycolipids containing a terminal α D-Gal-(1$\rightarrow$4)-D-Gal and purified globotriosyl ceramide (Gb_3), lyso-Gb_3 and hydatid cyst fluid have been used. In other ELISAs monoclonal antibodies against VT are used to bind toxin. In both types of assay bound toxin is detected with monoclonal or polyclonal antiserum against VT. These ELISAs are not as sensitive as Vero cell tests but are more rapid to perform. In addition, as VT toxins show variation in their antigenicity and binding, care must be taken in the choice of reagents if all VT producing strains are to be detected.

A.4.1.14 Use of DNA probes specific for VT genes will detect all VTEC and not only strains of serogroup O157. In addition to the polynucleotide probes for VT1 and VT2 derived from the cloned genes,[234, 235] synthetic oligonucleotide probes for the detection of different VT genes have also been developed.[211] The use of non-radioactively labelled probes for VT genes should enable these tests to be performed in a wider range of laboratories.[236] DNA probe tests can be performed using membranes with faecal blots or alternatively a large number of colonies from a sample or purified *E. coli* can be examined by hybridisation.

A.4.1.15 VT genes can also be detected by amplification in a polymerase chain reaction (PCR). The system first developed used 'degenerated primers' so that defined sequences of both VT1 and VT2 were amplified.[237] PCR products were identified by hybridization using specific oligonucleotide probes complementary to part of the amplified sequence. It was possible to identify VT1 or VT2 sequences but variants of VT2 could not be distinguished from VT2. Another PCR approach has been developed in which sets of primers were prepared for each VT gene defined so far (Table A.4.3). PCR tests can be performed on purified strains or preparations from faecal specimens. In order to reduce inhibition of amplification by components in faeces it is necessary to prepare DNA or alternatively wash the samples thoroughly before performing the PCR.

TABLE A.4.3

VT GENES

GENE DESIGNATION	GENE PRODUCT	REFERENCE
slt-I	VT1 or SLTI	Scotland *et al.*[238]
slt-II	VT2 or SLTII	O'Brien *et al.*[239]
slt-IIc	VT2v or SLTIIc	Scotland *et al.*[240] Schmitt *et al.*[241]
*vtx*2ha	VT2vha or SLTIIvha	Ito *et al.*[167]
*vtx*2hb	VT2vhb or SLTIIvhb	Ito *et al.*[167]
slt-IIv	VT2e, VTe or SLTIIv	Weinstein *et al.*[242]
slt-IIva	VT2ev, VTev or SLTIIva	Gannon *et al.*[168]

APPENDIX 4.2

SUB-TYPING METHODS FOR VTEC

Serotyping

A.4.2.1 Strains that have been confirmed as VTEC should be serotyped. This requires the facilities of a reference laboratory to test strains with antisera against 173 O antigens and 55 H antigens.[243] VT production has been reported in over 50 different O serogroups. Some VTEC belong to enteropathogenic O serogroups such as 26, 55, 111 and 128 and are detected by antisera for those serogroups which are commonly available in clinical laboratories.

Biotyping

A.4.2.2 Different biotypes of O157 VTEC with respect to fermentation patterns have been reported.[219] Most workers have considered the tests too irreproducible to be of use in the differentiation of this group.

'Phage typing

A.4.2.3 A 'phage typing scheme for O157 VTEC was developed in Canada for epidemiological investigations.[244] The scheme which uses 16 'phages has been extended in Canada and England and now recognizes over 80 types.[245, 246] (H. Lior personal communication). More than 20 'phage types have been identified in Britain but the majority of strains belong to types 1, 2, 4 and 49. This 'phage typing scheme is not used for VTEC of serogroups other than O157.

Plasmid analysis

A.4.2.4 Plasmid analysis of O157 VTEC can sometimes be used to identify strains in outbreaks and sporadic cases of infection.[182, 247] However this method is limited because virtually all O157 VTEC isolates carry a plasmid with a molecular weight of about 60×10^6, but some strains may carry additional plasmids.

VT gene analysis

A.4.2.5 Two major types of VT, VT1 and VT2, have been defined but several variants of VT2 have now been identified (Table A.4.3). The genes encoding these variants have been sequenced and this has led to the development of specific oligonucleotides that can be used as probes in DNA hybridization tests or primers in PCR amplification.[248, 249] Further differentiation of VT2 genes can be achieved by restriction fragment length polymorphism (RFLP) analysis of the amplification products. Alternatively, RFLP analysis with DNA probes can be performed using genomic DNA.[249]

Multilocus enzyme electrophoresis

A.4.2.6   Strains of O157 VTEC have been examined by multilocus enzyme electrophoresis. In a study by Whittam *et al.*,[250] genetic relatedness was estimated from allelic variation among 20 enzyme-encoding genes. Little variation was found in the O157:H7 strains and 95% of 369 strains belonged to a single electrophoretic type, ET11. The profiles of the closely related variant strains differed only by single alleles from that of ET11. It was also concluded that O157:H7 strains are most closely related to those of O55:H7.[250]

Pulsed-field gel electrophoresis

A.4.2.7   Pulsed-field gel electrophoresis (PFGE) of genomic DNA has been performed on O157 VTEC strains from different origins.[251, 252] In general, among the *E. coli* O157:H7 strains the restriction patterns were either identical or differed only by a few fragment bands. The enzymes found to be the most useful in these studies were *Xba*I and *Sfi*I. It was concluded that PFGE should be used together with other typing methods in epidemiological studies of O157 VTEC infections.[251]

'Phage λ probe analysis

A.4.2.8   Recently, a 'phage λ probe has been used in the analysis of genomic DNA from O157 VTEC.[104, 200] The RFLPs obtained with the λ -'phage probe differentiated the 72 strains into 23 groups. The use of λ-RFLPs together with toxin types and plasmid profiles provided further differentiation of O157 VTEC of human and bovine origin. A VT 'phage probe has also been used to examine O157 VTEC,[253] and this probe can subdivide strains within some of the common 'phage types such as PT2 and PT49.[15] It is recommended that a combination of methods should be used to allow maximal differentiation of O157 VTEC.

APPENDIX 4.3

SERODIAGNOSIS OF VTEC INFECTIONS

Antibodies to *E. coli* lipopolysaccharide (LPS)

A.4.3.1 Immunological tests have been developed to provide evidence of infection by *E. coli* O157; present tests use ELISA and immunoblotting. Patients with known O157 VTEC infection develop an increase in antibody titre to O157 LPS.[254] High titre serum antibodies to O157 LPS can also be detected in patients from which O157 VTEC have not been isolated. Control sera were negative for such antibodies.

A.4.3.2 Studies have been performed to examine responses to different Immunoglobulin (Ig) classes. Antibodies of the IgM class were demonstrated but patients with HUS caused by O157 VTEC did not produce antibodies of the IgG class to *E. coli* O157 LPS.[254] Some patients develop antibodies of the IgA class and the serum of some of these did not contain detectable IgM antibodies to *E. coli* O157 LPS.[38] Approximately 12% of cases developed IgA but not IgM antibodies to *E. coli* O157 LPS. A recent study in the United States also reported the presence of antibodies to *E. coli* O157 LPS but in this study 20 of 27 cases were positive for IgG.[255]

A.4.3.3 Cross reactions have been demonstrated between the LPS of *E. coli* O157 and the O antigen of other bacteria.[219, 256] Sera from patients with *E. coli* O157 react with the LPS of *Brucella abortus* and sera from brucellosis cases react with LPS of *E. coli* O157. Similarly, sera from patients infected with *Yersinia enterocolitica* O9 react with the LPS of *E. coli* O157 as well as the LPS of *Y. enterocolitica* O9. However, sera from patients with antibodies to *E. coli* O157 do not react with the LPS of *Y. enterocolitica* O9. The explanation for this one-way cross reaction is not clear. Further testing for cross reactions has shown that strains of *V. cholerae* O1 Inaba and group N *Salmonella* share epitopes with *E. coli* O157. Other cross reactions have been observed between *E. coli* O157 and some strains of *Escherichia hermannii* and *Citrobacter freundii*. These observations should be considered in the interpretation of serodiagnostic tests for *E. coli* O157.

A.4.3.4 Sera from cases of HUS have also been tested for the presence of antibodies to the LPS of VTEC belonging to serogroups other than O157.[257] Antibodies to the LPS of serogroups O5, O115, O145, O153 and O165 were demonstrated but in some patients no antibody response to the LPS of the infecting VTEC strain could be shown.

Antibodies to verocytotoxin

A.4.3.5 Early studies in Canada showed that patients with VTEC infection developed rising titres of VT neutralizing antibodies and this was used to diagnose VTEC infection in patients when other evidence was lacking.[179]

A.4.3.6   Other workers have investigated the ability of sera to neutralize the cytotoxic effects of VTs on tissue-culture cells. In a study in Britain sera from patients with diarrhoea or HUS and healthy adults were examined.[258] Sera from patients known to be infected by strains producing VT1 and VT2 did not have VT1 neutralizing activity although two sera from healthy adults did neutralize VT1. In contrast, VT2 neutralizing activity was found in most of the sera from patients and in all the sera from healthy adults. Studies in other laboratories have shown similar findings.[79, 180]   It has been suggested that factors other than immunoglobulins may cause the VT2 neutralizing activity.[259]

A.4.3.7   Sera from patients infected with O157 VTEC and healthy controls have been examined for immune responses to VT1 and VT2 by ELISA and immunoblotting. In a study in Britain, patients' sera could not be differentiated from control sera using ELISA and by immunoblotting none of the sera had antibodies to the A or B subunits of VT1 or VT2.[256] It was suggested that the concentrations of VT in patients may be too low to stimulate an immune response. In a Canadian study anti-VT1 IgG was detected by an ELISA. However, only a minority of HUS patients infected with VT1 producing strains developed anti-VT1 antibodies.[260]

A.4.3.8   Studies of sera in Germany for immunological responses to VT2 by immunoblot analysis and neutralizing activity showed reactivity by immunoblot in only 1 of 7 HUS patients and 11 of 260 healthy adults and children.[259] However, many sera had low VT2 - neutralizing activity but were immunoblot-negative. These results suggest that antibodies to VT2 are rarely produced and therefore, such tests have little diagnostic importance.

APPENDIX 5

EC AND UK LEGISLATION ON UNPASTEURISED COWS' MILK AND CREAM

General

A.5.1.1   The UK has recently implemented Directive 92/46/EEC,[261] which lays down rules for the production and marketing of raw milk, heat treated milk and milk based products. The Directive requires that all production holdings (dairy farms) should be registered and that milk treatment and processing establishments should be approved. There are also a range of other provisions including a requirement for hazard analysis procedures. Products made with raw milk have to be labelled as such for inspection purposes, although this does not apply at the retail level since the Directive does not extend to retail sales.

A.5.1.2   The Directive has been implemented in new national hygiene regulations - the Dairy Products (Hygiene) Regulations 1995.[262] These regulations were the subject of a public consultation exercise in Autumn 1994, and took effect from 9 May 1995. The regulations consolidate existing milk hygiene legislation contained in several statutory instruments. Certain national hygiene provisions (from existing national legislation) will be retained such as the time/temperature provisions for heat treated cream and ice-cream.

Provisions relating to raw drinking milk and cream

A.5.1.3   The Directive allows Member States to retain their national rules relating to the sale of raw milk or raw milk products by producers direct to consumers. In England and Wales current national controls on the production, distribution and labelling of untreated cows' milk (which are stricter than the requirements in the Directive) will be retained. The current national microbiological standard for untreated cows' milk is a Total Bacterial Count (TBC) not more than 20,000/ml and coliforms less than 100 per ml. In addition, the milk must carry a health warning and sales are restricted to the farm gate, farm catering outlets or distributors. Scotland will be continuing their ban on the sale of untreated cows' milk. In Northern Ireland there are similar arrangements to those in England and Wales.

A.5.1.4   In contrast to the sale of raw milk, raw cream is currently allowed to be sold without restrictions in England, Wales and Northern Ireland (but not Scotland), and this situation will continue under the new regulations as permitted under the Directive. However, EC microbiological standards will apply. Raw cows' milk intended for manufacture of raw cream will have to meet the following standards:

plate count at 30°C   (per ml) $\leq$ 100,000
somatic cell count   (per ml) $\leq$ 400,000
Staphylococcus aureus (per ml) n = 5, c = 2, m = 500, M = 2,000

Residues must also not exceed EC limits.

In addition, raw cream on removal from the processing establishment will have to meet the following standards:

Listeria monocytogenes	Absence in 1g
Salmonella spp.	Absence in 25g, where n = 5, c = 0

There is also a guideline (for use by manufacturers) for coliforms at 30°C.

Symbols referred to in the standards have the following meanings:

n = number of sample units comprising the sample;

c = number of sample units where the bacterial count may be between 'm' and 'M', the sample being considered acceptable if the bacterial count of the other sample units is 'm' or less;

m = threshold value for the number of bacteria, the result is considered satisfactory if the number of bacteria in all the sample units does not exceed 'm';

M = maximum value for the number of bacteria, the result is considered unsatisfactory if the number of bacteria in one or more sample units is 'M' or more.

REFERENCES

1. Kauffmann F. Review, The serology of the coli group. J. Immunol 1947; **57:** 71-100.

2. Neild G H. Haemolytic uraemic syndrome in practice. Lancet 1994; **343(8894):** 398-401.

3. Moake J L. Haemolytic uraemic syndrome: Basic science. Lancet 1994; **343(8894):** 393-397.

4. Griffin P M, Tauxe R V. The epidemiology of infections caused by *Escherichia coli* O157:H7, other enterohaemorrhagic *Escherichia coli*, and the associated haemolytic uraemic syndrome. Epidemiol Rev 1991; **13:** 60-98.

5. Thomas A, Chart H, Cheasty T, Smith H R, Frost J A, Rowe B. Verocytotoxin-producing *Escherichia coli*, particularly serogroup O157, associated with human infections in the United Kingdom: 1989-91. Epidemiol Infect 1993 Jun; **110(3):** 591-600.

6. Neill M A, Tarr P I, Clausen C R, Christie D L, Hickman R O. *Escherichia coli* O157:H7 as the predominant pathogen associated with the haemolytic uraemic syndrome: a prospective study in the Pacific Northwest. J Paediatr 1987 July; **80(1):** 37-40.

7. Taylor M. The haemolytic uraemic syndrome: a clinical perspective. PHLS Microbiol Digest 1990; **7(4):** 133-140.

8. Walters M D S, Matthei U, Kay R, Dillon M J, Barratt T M. The polymorphonuclear leucocyte count in childhood haemolytic uraemic syndrome. Paediatr Nephrol 1989; **3:** 130-134.

9. Karmali M A. Infection by Verocytotoxin-producing *Escherichia coli*. Clin Microbiol Rev 1989; **2:** 15-38.

10. Taylor C M, Milford D V, Rose P E, Roy T C F, Rowe B. The expression of blood group P1 in post-enteropathic haemolytic uraemic syndrome. Paediatr Nephrol 1990; **4:** 59-61.

11. Proulx F, Turgeon J P, Delage G, Lafleur L, Chicoine L. Randomised, controlled trial of antibiotic therapy for *Escherichia coli* O157:H7 enteritis. J Paediatr 1992; **121(2):** 299-303.

12. PHLS Interim Guidelines for the control of infections with Verocytotoxin-producing *Escherichia coli* (VTEC). CDR. In press.

13. Department of Health. Management of Outbreaks of Foodborne Illness: Guidance Produced by a Department of Health Working Group, 1994.

14. United States Department of Agriculture, Food Safety and Inspection Service, May 21, 1993. Report on the *Escherichia coli* O157:H7 outbreak in the Western States.

15. Willshaw G A, Thirlwell J, Jones A P, Parry S, Salmon R L, Hickey M. Verocytotoxin-producing *Escherichia coli* O157 in beefburgers linked to an outbreak of diarrhoea, haemorrhagic colitis and haemolytic uraemic syndrome in Britain. Lett Appl Microbiol 1994; **19(5):** 304-307.

16. Burnens A P, Zbinden R, Kaempf L, Heinzer I, Nicolet J. A case of laboratory acquired infection with *Escherichia coli* O157: H7. Zbl Bakt 1993; **279:** 512-517.

17. Konowalchuk J, Spiers J I, Stavric S. Vero response to a cytotoxin of *Escherichia coli*. Infect Immun 1977; **18(3):** 775-779.

18. Tesh V L, Samuel J E, Perera L P, Sharefkin J B, O'Brien A D. Evaluation of the role of Shiga and Shiga-like toxins in mediating direct damage to human vascular endothelial cells. J Infect Dis 1991; **164:** 344-352.

19. Strockbine N A, Jackson M P, Sung L M, Holmes R K, O'Brien A D. Cloning and sequencing of the genes for Shiga toxin from *Shigella dysenteriae* type 1. J Bacteriol 1988; **170:** 1116-1122.

20. Strockbine N A, Marques L R M, Newland J W, Smith H W, Holmes R K, O'Brien A D. Two toxin-converting 'phages from *Escherichia coli* O157:H7 strain 933 encode antigenically distinct toxins with similar biological activities. Infect Immun 1986; **53(1):** 135-140.

21. Smith H R, Scotland S M. Methods to provide evidence of infection by Verocytotoxin-producing *Escherichia coli*. PHLS Microbiol Digest 1990; **7(4):** 128-132.

22. Richardson S E, Rotman T A, Jay V, Smith C R, Becker L E, Petric M, Olivieri N F, Karmali M A. Experimental Verocytotoxemia in rabbits. Infect Immun 1992; **60:** 4154-4167.

23. Richardson S E, Karmali M A, Becker L E, Smith C R. The histopathology of the haemolytic uraemic syndrome associated with Verocytotoxin-producing *Escherichia coli* infections. Human Path 1988; **19:** 1102-1108.

24. Chart H, Law D, Rowe B, Acheson D W K. Patients with haemolytic uraemic syndrome caused by *Escherichia coli* O157: absence of antibodies to Verocytotoxin 1 (VT1) or VT2. J Clin Path 1993; **46:** 1053-1054.

25. Obrig T G, Del Vecchio P J, Brown J E, Moran T P, Rowland B M, Judge T K, *et al.* Direct cytotoxic action of Shiga toxin on human vascular endothelial cells. Infect Immun 1988; **56:** 2373-2378.

26. Louie C B, Obrig T G. Shiga toxin-associated haemolytic-uraemic syndrome: combined cytotoxic effects of Shiga toxin, interleukin-1 B, and tumour necrosis factor alpha on human vascular endothelial cells *in vitro*. Infect Immun 1991; **59:** 4173-4179.

27. Pearson G R, Watson C A, Hall G A, Wray C. Natural infection with an attaching and effacing *Escherichia coli* in the small and large intestines of a calf with diarrhoea. Vet Rec 1989; **124:** 297-299.

28. Wray C, McLaren I, Pearson G R. Occurrence of attaching and effacing lesions in the small intestine of calves experimentally infected with bovine isolates of Verotoxigenic *Escherichia coli*. Vet Rec 1989; **125:** 365-368.

29. Moxley R A, Francis D H. Natural and experimental infection with an attaching and effacing strain of *Escherichia coli* in calves. Infect Immun 1986; **53(2):** 339-346.

30. Francis D H, Collins J E, Duimstra J R. Infection of gnotobiotic pigs with an *Escherichia coli* O157:H7 strain associated with an outbreak of haemorrhagic colitis. Infect Immun 1986; **51(3):** 953-956.

31. Salmon R L, Smith R M M. How common is *Escherichia coli* O157, and where is it coming from? Total population surveillance in Wales 1990-1993. Second International Symposium and Workshop on Verocytotoxin (Shiga-like)-producing *Escherichia coli* infections [abstract no. P1.55]; 1994 June 27-30; Bergamo, Italy.

32. Hall S M, Banks J, Marshall R. Survey of *Escherichia coli* O157. PHLS Microbiol Digest 1990; **7(4):** 152-153.

33. Steering Group on the Microbiological Safety of Food. Report of Progress 1990-1992. London: HMSO 1993.

34. Taylor C M, Milford D V, White R H. A plea for standardised technology within the haemolytic uraemic syndromes. Paediatr Nephrol 1991 Jan; **5(1):** 97.

35. Coad N A, Marshall T, Rowe B, Taylor C M. Changes in the post-enteropathic form of the haemolytic uraemic syndrome in children. Clin Nephrol 1991 Jan; **35(1):** 10-6.

36. Abu-Arafeh I A, Smail P J, Youngson G G, Auchterlonie I A. Haemolytic uraemic syndrome in the defined population of northeast of Scotland. Euro J Paediatr 1991 Feb; **150(4):** 279-281.

37.   Milford D V, Taylor C M, Gutteridge B, Hall S M, Rowe B, Kleanthous H. Haemolytic uraemic syndromes in the British Isles 1985-88: association with Verocytotoxin-producing *Escherichia coli*. Part 1: Clinical and epidemiological aspects. Archives of Disease in Childhood 1990 Jul; **65(7):** 716-721.

38.   Chart H, Rowe B. Improved detection of infection by *Escherichia coli* O157 in patients with haemolytic syndrome by means of IgA antibodies to lipopolysaccharide. J Infect 1992; **24(3):** 257-261.

39.   Ashkenazi S, May L, LaRocco M, Lopez E L, Cleary T G. The effect of postnatal age on the adherence of enterohaemorrhagic *Escherichia coli* to rabbit intestinal cells. Paediatric Res 1991 Jan; **26(1):** 14-19.

40.   Fitzpatrick M M, Shah V, Trompeter R S, Dillon M J, Barratt T M. Long term renal outcome of childhood haemolytic uraemic syndrome. Brit Med J 1991; **303(6801):** 489-492.

41.   Trompeter R S, Schwartz R, Chantler C, Dillon M J, Haycock G B, Kay R, *et al*. Haemolytic uraemic syndrome: An analysis of prognostic features. Archives of Disease in Childhood 1983 Feb; **58(2):** 101-105.

42.   Surveillance of haemolytic uraemic syndrome 1983-4: British Paediatric Association-Communicable Disease Surveillance Centre. Brit Med J 1986; **292(6513):** 115-117.

43.   Haemolytic Uraemic Syndrome Surveillance: British Paediatric Surveillance Unit/CDSC Surveillance Scheme. CDR Weekly 1990; **90/21:** 1.

44.   Kohli H S, Chandhuri A K R, Todd W T A, Mitchell A A B, Liddell K G. The Hartwoodhill Hospital *Escherichia coli* O157 outbreak. Communicable Diseases and Environmental Health in Scotland Weekly Report 1993; **27:** (93/13), 8-11.

45.   Morgan G M, Newman C, Palmer S R. First recognised community outbreak of haemorrhagic colitis due to Verocytotoxin-producing *Escherichia coli* O157 in the UK. Epidemiol Infect 1988; **101:** 83-91.

46.   Salmon R L, Farrell I D, Hutchinson J G, Coleman D J, Gross R J, Fry N K, *et al*. A christening party outbreak of haemorrhagic colitis and haemolytic uraemic syndrome associated with *Escherichia coli* O157:H7. Epidemiol Infect 1989 Oct; **103(2):** 249-254.

47.   Chapman P A, Wright D J, Higgins R. Untreated milk as a source of Verotoxigenic *Escherichia coli*. Vet Rec 1993; **133(7):** 171-172.

48.   Morgan D, Newman C P, Hutchinson D N, Walker A M, Rowe B, Masid F. Verocytotoxin-producing *Escherichia coli* O157 infections associated with the consumption of yoghurt. Epidemiol Infect 1993; **111:** 181-187.

49. Brewster D H, Brown M I, Robertson D, Houghton G L, Brinson J, Sharp J C M. An outbreak of *Escherichia coli* O157 associated with a children's paddling pool. Epidemiol Infect 1994; **112:** 441-447.

50. Upton P, Coia J E. Outbreak of *Escherichia coli* O157 infection associated with pasteurised milk supply [letter]. Lancet 1994; **344(8928):** 1015.

51. Belongia E A, Osterholm M T, Soler J T, Ammend D A, Braun J E, MacDonald K L. Transmission of *Escherichia coli* O157:H7 infection in Minnesota child day-care facilities. J Amer Med Assoc 1993 Feb 17; **269(7):** 883-888.

52. Lopez E L, Diaz M, Devoto S, Grinstein S, Woloj M, Murray B E, *et al.* Evidence of infection with organisms producing Shiga-like toxins in household contacts of children with haemolytic uraemic syndrome. Paediatr Infect Dis J 1991 Jan; **10(1):** 20-24.

53. Booth L, Rowe B. Possible occupational acquisition of *Escherichia coli* O157 infection. Lancet 1993; **342(8882):** 1298-1299.

54. Riley L W, Remis R S, Helgerson S D. Haemorrhagic colitis associated with a rare *Escherichia coli* serotype. New Engl J Med 1983; **308:** 681-685.

55. Hockin J, Lior H, Stratton F. Haemorrhagic colitis due to *Escherichia coli* (Verotoxigenic) in Canada. Can Dis Weekly Rep 1988; **14:** 147-148.

56. Griffin P M, Tauxe R V. *Escherichia coli* O157:H7 human illness in North America, food vehicles and animal reservoirs. Intern Food Safety News 1993; **2:** 2.

57. Tarr P I, Neill M A, Clausen C R, Watkins S L, Christie D L, Hickman R O. *Escherichia coli* O157:H7 and the haemolytic uraemic syndrome: Importance of early cultures in establishing the etiology. J Infect Dis 1990; **162(2):** 553-556.

58. Griffin P M, Ries A A, Greene K D. *Escherichia coli* O157:H7 diarrhoea in the US: a multi-centre surveillance project. 80th meeting of the International Association of Milk, Food and Environmental Sanitarians; 1993 Aug 1-4; Atlanta, Georgia, USA.

59. Ostroff S M, Kobayashi J M, Lewis J H. Infections with *Escherichia coli* O157:H7 in Washington State. The first year of statewide disease surveillance. J Amer Med Assoc 1989; **262:** 355-359.

60. Pai C H, Ahmed N, Lior H. Epidemiology of sporadic diarrhoea due to Verocytotoxin-producing *Escherichia coli*: a two year prospective study. J Infect Dis 1988; **157:** 1054-1057.

61. Griffin P M. *E. coli* O157:H7 and other enterohaemorrhagic *E. coli* In: Blaser M J, Greenberg H B, Guerrant R L, editors. Infections of the gastrointestinal tract, 1995. [in press]

62. Wells J G, Davis B R, Wachsmuth I K, Riley L W, Remis R S, Sokolow R, *et al.* Laboratory investigation of haemorrhagic colitis outbreaks associated with a rare *Escherichia coli* serotype. J Clin Microbiol 1983; **18:** 512-520.

63. Belongia E A, MacDonald K L, Parham G L, White K E, Korlath J A, Lobato M N, *et al.* An outbreak of *Escherichia coli* O157:H7 colitis associated with consumption of pre-cooked meat patties. J Infect Dis 1991; **164:** 338-343.

64. Martin M L, Shipman L D, Wells J G. Isolation of *Escherichia coli* O157:H7 from dairy cattle associated with two cases of haemolytic uraemic syndrome. Lancet 1986; **II(8514):** 1043.

65. Wells J G, Shipman L D, Greene K D, Sowers E G, Green J H, Cameron D N, *et al.* Isolation of *Escherichia coli* serotype O157:H7 and other shiga-like toxin producing *Escherichia coli* from dairy cattle. J Clin Microbiol 1991; **29(5):** 985-989.

66. Holton D. Overview of the epidemiology of VTEC disease in Canada. In: Todd E C D, MacKenzie J M, editors. Proceedings of a workshop on methods to isolate *Escherichia coli* O157:H7 and other Verotoxigenic *Escherichia coli* in foods, Ottawa, Canada, 1991 Mar 18-19. Polyscience Publications Inc. 1993: 1-12.

67. Rowe P C, Orrbine E, Ogborn M, Wells G A, Winther W, Lior H, *et al.* Epidemic *Escherichia coli* O157:H7 gastroenteritis and haemolytic uraemic syndrome in a Canadian Inuit community: Intestinal illness in family members as a risk factor. J Paediatr 1994; **124:** 21-26.

68. Swerdlow D L, Woodruff B A, Brady R C, Griffin P M, Tippen S, Donnell H D, *et al.* A waterborne outbreak in Missouri of *Escherichia coli* O157:H7 associated with bloody diarrhoea and death. Ann Intern Med 1992; **117:** 812-819.

69. Besser R E, Lett S M, Weber J T, Doyle M P, Barrett T S, Wells J G, *et al.* An outbreak of diarrhoea and haemolytic uraemic syndrome from *Escherichia coli* O157:H7 in fresh-pressed apple cider. J Amer Med Assoc 1993; **269(17):** 2217-2220.

70. Keene W E, McAnulty J M, Williams L P, Huesly F C, Hedberg K, Fleming D W. A two-restaurant outbreak of *Escherichia coli* O157:H7 enteritis associated with the consumption of mayonnaise. Program and Abstracts of the Interscience Conference on Antimicrobial Agents and Chemotherapy. 1993; **33:** 354.

71. Weagant S D, Bryant J L, Bark D H. Survival of *Escherichia coli* O157:H7 in mayonnaise-based sauces at room and refrigerated temperatures. J Food Protect 1994; **57(7):** 629-631.

72. Cieslak P R, Barrett T J, Griffin P M. *Escherichia coli* O157:H7 infection from a manured garden. Lancet 1993; **342(8867):** 367.

73.   MacDonald K L, O'Leary M J, Cohen M L. *Escherichia coli* O157:H7, an emerging gastrointestinal pathogen. Results of a one-year prospective population based study. J Amer Med Assoc 1988; **259:** 3567-3570.

74.   Bryant H E, Athar M A, Pai C H. Risk factors for *Escherichia coli* O157:H7 infection in an urban community. J Infect Dis 1989; **160:** 858-864.

75.   Tarr P I. *Escherichia coli* O157:H7 outbreak in the Western United States. The 80th Annual Meeting of the Association of Milk, Food and Environmental Sanitarians [abstract]; 1993 Aug 1-4; Atlanta, Georgia, USA.

76.   Tarr P I. Review of 1993 *Escherichia coli* O157:H7 outbreak in the Western United States. Dairy Food Environ Sanit 1994; **14(7):** 372-373.

77.   Turney C, Green-Smith M, Shipp M, Mordhorst C, Whittingslow C, Brawley L, *et al*. *Escherichia coli* O157:H7 outbreak linked to home-cooked hamburger - California, July 1993. Morbidity and Mortality Weekly Report 1994 **43(12):**213-216.

78.   World Health Organisation. Surveillance Programme for Control of Foodborne Infections and Intoxications in Europe, Fifth Report 1985-1989. Institute of Veterinary Medicine - Robert von Ostertag Institute (FAO/WHO Collaborating Centre for Research and Training in Food Hygiene and Zoonoses), Berlin, 1992.

79.   Bitzan M, Ludwig K, Klemt M, Konig H, Buren J, Muller-Wiefel D E. The role of *Escherichia coli* O157 infections in the classical (enteropathic) haemolytic uraemic syndrome: results of a Central European multicentre study. Epidemiol Infect 1993; **110:** 183-196.

80.   Mariani-Kurkdjian P, Ranamur E, Milton A, Picard B, Lane H, Lambert-Zechovsky N, *et al*. Identification of a clone of *Escherichia coli* O103:H2 as a potential agent of HUS in France. J Clin Microbiol 1993; **31(2):** 296-301.

81.   Two clusters of haemolytic uraemic syndrome in France. CDR Weekly Report 1994 Feb; **4(7):** 1.

82.   Pierard D, Stevens S, Morian L, Lior H, Lammers S. Three years PCR screening for VTEC in human starts in Brussels. Proceedings of Second International Symposium and Workshop on Verocytotoxin (Shiga-like toxin) - producing *Escherichia coli* infections [abstract no.01.4]; 1994 June Bergamo, Italy.

83.   Caprioli A, Luzzi I, Minelli F, Tozzi A E, Niccolini A, Gianviti A, *et al*. Haemolytic uraemic syndrome and Verocytotoxin-producing *Escherichia coli* infections in Italy. Proceedings of the 2nd International Symposium and Workshop in Verocytotoxin (Shiga-like) - producing *Escherichia coli* infections [abstract no.01.3]; 1994 June; Bergamo, Italy.

84.   Wray C, McLaren I M, Carroll P J. *Escherichia coli* isolated from farm animals in England and Wales between 1986 and 1991. Vet Rec 1993; **133:** 439-442.

85.   Chanter N, Hall G A, Bland A P, Hayle A J, Parsons K R. Dysentery in calves caused by an atypical strain of *Escherichia coli.* Vet Microbiol 1986; **12(3):** 241-254.

86.   Schoonderwoerd M, Clarke R C, Van-Dreumel A A, Rawluk S A. Colitis in calves: natural and experimental infection with a Verocytotoxin-producing strain of *Escherichia coli* O111:NM. Can J Vet Res 1988; **52:** 484-487.

87.   Mainil J G, Duchesnes C J, Whipp S C, Marques L R M, O'Brien A D, Casey T A, *et al.* Shiga-like toxin production and attaching and effacing activity of *Escherichia coli* associated with calf diarrhoea. Amer J Vet Res 1987; **48:** 743-748.

88.   Orskov F, Orskov I, Villar J A. Cattle as a reservoir of Verocytotoxin-producing *Escherichia coli* O157:H7. Lancet 1987; **II(8553):** 276.

89.   Smith H R, Scotland S M, Willshaw G A, Wray C, McLaren I M, Cheasty T, *et al.* Verocytotoxin production and presence of VT genes in *Escherichia coli* strains of animal origin. J Gen Microbiol 1988; **134:** 829-834.

90.   Gonzalez E A, Blanco J. Serotypes and antibiotic resistance of Verotoxigenic (VTEC) and necrotising (NTEC) *Escherichia coli* strains isolated from calves with diarrhoea. FEMS Microbiol Lett 1989; **60:** 31-36.

91.   Scotland S, Willshaw G A, Smith H R, Rowe B. Properties of strains of *Escherichia coli* O26:H11 in relation to their enteropathogenic or enterohaemorrhagic classification. J Infect Dis 1990; **162:** 1069-1074.

92.   Montenegro M A, Bulte M, Trumpf T, Aleksic S, Reuter G, Bulling E, *et al.* Detection and characterisation of faecal Verocytotoxin-producing *Escherichia coli* from healthy cattle. J. Clin Microbiol 1990; **28:** 1417-1421.

93.   Wilson J B, McEwen S A, Clarke R C, Leslie K E, Wilson R A, Waltner-Toews D, *et al.* Distribution and characteristics of Verocytotoxigenic *Escherichia coli* isolated from Ontario dairy cattle. Epidemiol Infect 1992; **108:** 423-439.

94.   Chapman P A, Siddons C A, Wright D J, Norman P, Fox J, Crick E. Cattle as a source of Verotoxigenic *Escherichia coli* O157. Vet Rec 1992; **131(14):** 323-324.

95.   Read S C, Gyles C L, Clarke R C, Lior H, McEwan S. Prevalence of Verocytotoxigenic *Escherichia coli* in minced beef, pork and chicken in southwestern Ontario. Epidemiol Infect 1990; **105:** 11-20.

96.   Smith H R, Cheasty T, Roberts D, Thomas A, Rowe B. Examination of retail chickens and sausages in Britain for Verocytotoxin-producing *Escherichia coli.* Appl Environ Microbiol 1991; **57:** 2091-2093.

97. Willshaw G A, Scotland S M, Smith H R, Rowe B. Properties of Verocytotoxin-producing *Escherichia coli* of human origin of O serogroups other than O157. J Infect Dis 1992; **166:** 797-802.

98. Borczyk A A, Karmali M A, Lior H, Duncan L M C. Bovine reservoir for Verocytotoxin-producing *Escherichia coli* O157:H7. Lancet 1987; **I(8524):** 98.

99. Padhye N V, Doyle M P. *Escherichia coli* O157:H7: epidemiology, pathogenesis and methods of detection in food. J Food Protect 1992; **55:** 555-565.

100. Smith H R, Rowe B, Gross R J, Fry N K, Scotland S M. Haemorrhagic colitis and Verocytotoxin-producing *Escherichia coli* in England and Wales. Lancet 1987; **I(8541):** 1062-1064.

101. Chapman P A, Wright D J, Norman P. Verocytotoxin-producing *Escherichia coli* infections in Sheffield: cattle as a possible source. Epidem Infect 1989; **102:** 439-455.

102. Chapman P A, Siddons C A, Wright D J, Norman P, Fox J, Crick E. Cattle as a possible source of Verocytotoxin-producing *Escherichia coli* O157 infections in man. Epidemiol Infect 1993; **111(3):** 439-447.

103. Chapman P A, Siddons C A. A comparison of strains of *Escherichia coli* O157 from humans and cattle in Sheffield, England. J Infect Dis 1994; **170:** 251-252.

104. Paros M, Tarr P I, Kim H, Besser T E, Hancock D D. A comparison of human and bovine *Escherichia coli* O157:H7 isolates by toxin genotype, plasmid profile and bacteriophage λ-restriction fragment length polymorphism profile. J Infect Dis 1993; **168:** 1300-1303.

105. Clarke R S, McEwen S, Harnett N, Lior H, Gyles C. The prevalence of Verotoxin-producing *Escherichia coli* (VTEC) in bovines at slaughter. Abstr Ann Meet Amer Soc Microbiol 1988; **88:** 282.

106. United States Department of Agriculture, *Escherichia coli* O157:H7 in US Dairy Calves. National Animal Health Monitoring System. Centers for Epidemiology and Animal Health. 555 South Howes, Suite 200, Fort Collins, Colorado, USA, 1994 Jan.

107. Hancock D D. Establishment of a bovine surveillance programme for *Escherichia coli* O157:H7 in Washington State. 80th meeting of the International Association of Milk, Food and Environmental Sanitarians, Atlanta, Georgia, USA, 1993 Aug 1-4.

108. Hancock D D. Food Safety from Farm to Table, *Escherichia coli* O157:H7 - A two day conference sponsored by Washington State University - 27 December 1993. Population Medicine News 1993; **6(12):** 1-16.

109. Synge B A, Hopkins G F. Studies of Verocytotoxic *Escherichia coli* O157:H7 in cattle in Scotland and association with human outbreaks. Proceedings of Second International Symposium and Workshop on Verocytotoxin (Shiga-like toxin) - producing *Escherichia coli* infections [abstract no. P1.14]; 1994 June; Bergamo, Italy.

110. The Microbiological Safety of Food: Part II. Report of the Committee on the Microbiological Safety of Food (Chairman: Sir Mark Richmond). London: HMSO, 1991.

111. Council Directive 91/497/EEC, Official J No. L087 02.04.92

112. Council Directive 64/433/EEC, Official J No. L121 29.07.64

113. Council Directive 92/5/EEC, Official J No. L57 02.03.92.

114. Council Directive 77/99/EEC, Official J No. L26 31.01.77.

115. The Meat Products (Hygiene) Regulations. S I No. 3082. London: HMSO 1994.

116. Council Directive 88/657/EEC, Official J No. L382 31.12.88.

117. Council Directive 94/65/EC, Official J No. L12 15.01.94.

118. Dickson J S, Anderson M E. Microbial decontamination of food animal carcases by washing and sanitizing systems: a review. J Food Protect 1992; **55(2):** 133-140.

119. Willshaw G A, Smith H R, Roberts D, Thirlwell J, Cheasty T, Rowe B. Examination of raw beef products for the presence of Verocytotoxin-producing *Escherichia coli*, particularly those of serogroup O157. J Appl Bacteriol. 1993; **75:** 420-426.

120. Neaves P, Deacon J, Bell C. A survey of the incidence of *Escherichia coli* O157 in the UK Dairy Industry. Int Dairy J 1994; **4:** 679-696.

121. Samadpour M, Ongerty J E, Listen J, Tran N, Nguyen D, Whitlam T S, *et al.* Occurrence of shiga-like toxin-producing *Escherichia coli* in retail fresh seafood, beef, lamb, pork and poultry from grocery stores in Seattle, Washington. Appl Environ Microbiol 1994; **60(3):** 1038-1040.

122. Suthienkul O, Brown J E, Seriwatana J, Tienthongdee S, Sastravaha S, Echeverria P. Shiga-like toxin-producing *Escherichia coli* in retail meats and cattle in Thailand. Appl Environ Microbiol 1990; **56(4):** 1135-1139.

123. Doyle M P, Schoeni S L. Isolation of *Escherichia coli* O157:H7 from retail fresh meats and poultry. Appl Environ Microbiol 1987; **53:** 2394-2396.

124. Padhye N V, Doyle M P. Rapid procedure for detecting enterohaemorrhagic *Escherichia coli* O157:H7 in food. Appl Environ Microbiol 1991; **57(9):** 2693-2698.

125. Bowen D A, Henning D R. Coliform bacteria and *Staphylococcus aureus* in retail natural cheeses. J Food Protect 1994; **57(3)**: 253-255.

126. Sekla L, Milley D, Stakiw W, Sisler J, Drew J, Sargent D. Verocytotoxin-producing *Escherichia coli* in ground beef - Manitoba. Can Dis Weekly Rep 1990 June 2; **16(22)**: 103-105.

127. Food MicroModel User Manual. Food MicroModel Ltd, Leatherhead: 1994.

128. Doyle M P, Schoeni S L. Survival and growth characteristics of *Escherichia coli* associated with haemorrhagic colitis. Appl Environ Microbiol 1984; **48(4)**: 855-856.

129. Milley D G, Sekla L H. An enzyme-linked immunosorbent assay-based isolation procedure for verotoxigenic *Escherichia coli*. Appl Environ Microbiol 1993; **59(12)**: 4223-4229.

130. Alcock S J. Growth characteristics of food poisoning organisms at sub-optimal temperatures. Campden Food and Drink Research Association, Chipping Campden, Gloucestershire, England; 1987. Technical Memo. No.: 440.

131. Davies A R, Slade A, Blood R M, Gibbs P A. Effect of temperature and pH value on the growth of verotoxigenic *E. coli*. Leatherhead Food Research Association. 1992. Research Report No.: 691.

132. Elliott R P. Temperature-gradient incubator for determining the temperature range of growth of micro-organisms. J Bacteriol 1963; **85**: 889-894.

133. Zhao T, Doyle M P, Besser R E. Fate of enterohaemorrhagic *Escherichia coli* O157:H7 in apple cider with and without preservatives. Appl Environ Microbiol 1993; **59(8)**: 2526-2530.

134. Abdul-Raouf U M, Beuchat L R, Ammar M S. Survival and growth of *Escherichia coli* O157:H7 on salad vegetables. Appl Environ Microbiol 1993; **59(7)**: 1999-2006.

135. Betts G D, Lyndon G, Brooks J. Heat resistance of emerging foodborne pathogens: *Aeromonas hydrophila, Escherichia coli* O157:H7, *Plesiomonas shigelloides* and *Yersinia enterocolitica*. Campden Food and Drink Research Association, Chipping Campden, Gloucestershire, England; 1993. Technical Memo No.: 672.

136. D'Aoust J Y, Park C E, Szabo R A, Todd E C D, Emmons D B, Mckellar R C. Thermal inactivation of *Campylobacter* species, *Yersinia enterocolitica* and haemorrhagic *Escherichia coli* O157:H7 in fluid milk. J Dairy Sci 1988; **71**: 3230-3236.

137. Arocha M M, McVey M, Loder, S D, Rupnow J H, Bullerman L. Behaviour of haemorrhagic *Escherichia coli* O157:H7 during the manufacture of cottage cheese. J Food Protect 1992; **55(5)**: 379-381.

138. Murano E A, Pierson M D. Effect of heat shock and growth atmosphere on the heat resistance of *Escherichia coli* O157:H7. J Food Protect 1992; **55(3):** 171-175.

139. Todd E, Hughes A, Mackenzie J, Caldeira R, Gleeson T, Brown B. Thermal resistance of verotoxigenic *Escherichia coli* in ground beef - initial work. In: Todd E C D, MacKenzie J M editors. Proceedings of a workshop on methods to isolate *Escherichia coli* O157:H7 and other Verotoxigenic *Escherichia coli* in foods, Ottawa, Canada, 1991 Mar 18-19. Polyscience Publications Inc. 1993: 93-110.

140. Line J E, Fain A R, Moran A B, Martin L M, Lechowich R V, Carosella J M, *et al.* Lethality of heat to *Escherichia coli* O157:H7: D-value and z-value determinations in ground beef. J Food Protect 1991; **54(10):** 762-766.

141. Glass K A, Loeffelholz J H, Ford J P, Doyle M P. Fate of *Escherichia coli* O157:H7 as affected by pH or sodium chloride and in fermented, dry sausage. Appl Environ Microbiol 1992; **58:** 2513-2516.

142. Conner D E. Temperature and NaCl affects growth and survival of *Escherichia coli* O157:H7 in poultry-based and laboratory media. J Food Sci 1992; **57:** 532-533.

143. Abdul-Raouf U M, Beuchat L R, Ammar M S. Survival and growth of *Escherichia coli* O157:H7 in ground roasted beef as affected by pH, acidulants and temperature. Appl Environ Microbiol 1993; **59(8):** 2364-2368.

144. Miller, L G, Kaspar C W. *Escherichia coli* O157:H7 acid tolerance and survival in apple cider. J Food Protect 1994; **57(6):** 460-464.

145. Thayer D N, Boyd G. Elimination of *Escherichia coli* O157:H7 in meats by gamma irradiation. Appl Environ Microbiol 1993; **59:** 1030-1034.

146. Clavero M R S, Monk J D, Beucht L R, Doyle M P, Brackett R E. Inactivation of *Escherichia coli* O157:H7, Salmonellae and *Campylobacter jejuni* in raw ground beef by gamma irradiation. Appl Environ Microbiol 1994; **60(6):** 2069-2075.

147. Thomas L V, Wimpenny J W T, Davis S G. Effect of three preservatives on the growth of *Bacillus cereus*, Verocytotoxigenic *Escherichia coli* and *Staphylococcus aureus* on plates with gradients of pH and sodium chloride concentration. Int J Food Microbiol 1993; **17(4):** 289-301.

148. Buchanan R L, Klawitter L A. The effect of incubation temperature, initial pH and sodium chloride on the growth kinetics of *Escherichia coli* O157:H7. Food Microbiol 1992; **9:** 185-196.

149. Advisory Committee on the Microbiological Safety of Food: Interim Report on *Campylobacter*. London: HMSO, 1993.

150. Campden Food and Drink Research Association. HACCP: A practical guide, Chipping Campden, Gloucestershire, England; 1992. Technical Manual No.: 38.

151. World Health Organisation. Division of Food and Nutrition Food Safety Unit: Training Considerations for the Application of the Hazard Analysis Critical Control Point System to Food Processing and Manufacturing, 1993.

152. International Commission on Microbiological Specifications for Foods (ICMSF). Microorganisms in Foods, 4. Application of the Hazard Analysis Critical Control Point (HACCP) system to ensure microbiological safety and quality. Blackwell Scientific Publications, Ltd., Oxford, 1988.

153. Department of Health. Assured Safe Catering. A Management System for Hazard Analysis. London: HMSO, 1993.

154. Sockett P N. Communicable disease associated with milk and dairy products: England and Wales 1987-1989. CDR Rev 1991; **1(1):** 9-12.

155. Department of Health. Safer Cooked Meat Production Guidelines. A 10 Point Plan. London 1992.

156. Ministry of Agriculture, Fisheries and Food. Food Safety [leaflet]. London: Foodsense, 1994.

157. United States Department of Agriculture, Food Safety and Inspection Service: Heat Processing, Cooking and Cooling, Handling and Storage Requirements for Uncured Meat Patties (9 CFR Parts 318 and 320). Federal Register 1993 Aug; **58(156):** 41138-41152.

158. United States Department of Health and Human Services, Food Code 1993, Public Health Service, Food and Drug Administration, Washington. 1994; 50-60.

159. Hague M A, Warren K E, Hunt M C, Kropf D H, Kastner C L, Stroda S L, *et al.* Endpoint temperature, internal cooked colour, and expressible juice colour relationships in ground beef patties. J Food Sci 1994; **59(3):** 465-470.

160. Department of Health. Chilled and Frozen. Guidelines on Cook-Chill and Cook-Freeze Catering Systems. London: HMSO, 1989.

161. Tesh V L, O'Brien A D. Adherence and colonization mechanisms of enteropathogenic and enterohaemorrhagic *Escherichia coli*. Microbiol Pathogen 1992; **12:** 245-254.

162. Jackson M P. Structure-function analyses of Shiga toxin and the Shiga-like toxins. Microbial Pathogen 1990; **8:** 235-242.

163. Sherman P M , Soni R. Adherence of Verocytotoxin-producing *Escherichia coli* of serotype O157:H7 to human epithelial cells in tissue-culture: role of outer membranes as bacterial adhesins. J Med Microbiol 1988; **26:** 11-17.

164. Marques L R H, Peiris J S M. Cryz S J, O'Brien A D. *Escherichia coli* strains isolated from pigs with edema disease produce a variant of Shiga-like toxin II. FEMS Microbiol Lett 1987; **44:** 33-38.

165. Tesh V L, O'Brien A D. The pathogenic mechanisms of Shiga toxins and the Shiga-like toxins. Molecular Microbiol 1991; **5:** 1817-1822.

166. Jackson M P, Neill R J, O'Brien A D, Holmes R K, Newland J W. Nucleotide sequence analysis and comparison of the structural genes for Shiga-like toxin I and Shiga-like toxin II encoded by bacteriophages from *Escherichia coli* 933. FEMS Microbiol Lett 1987; **44:** 109-114.

167. Ito H, Terai A, Kurazono H, Takeda Y, Nishibuchi M. Cloning and nucleotide sequencing of Verocytotoxin 2 variant genes from *Escherichia coli* O91:H21 isolated from a patient with the haemolytic uraemic syndrome. Microbiol Pathogen 1990; **8:** 47-60.

168. Gannon V P J, Teerling C, Masri S A, Gyles C L. Molecular cloning and nucleotide sequence of another variant of the *Escherichia coli* Shiga-like toxin II family. J Gen Microbiol 1990; **136:** 1125-1135.

169. O'Brien A D, Holmes R K. Shiga and Shiga-like toxins. Microbiol Rev 1987; **51:** 206-220.

170. Calderwood S B, Acheson D W K. A system for production and rapid purification of large amounts of Shiga toxin/Shiga-like toxin IB subunit. Infect Immun 1990; **58:** 2977-2982.

171. Jacewicz M, Clausen H, Nudelman E, Donohue-Rolfe A, Keusch G T. Pathogenesis of *Shigella* diarrhoea XI. Isolation of *Shigella* toxin-binding glycolipid from rabbit jejunum and HeLa cells and its identification as globotriaosylceramide. J Exp Med 1986; **163:** 1391-1404.

172. Lingwood C A, Law H, Richardson S, Martin P, Brunton J L, De Grandis S, *et al.* Glycolipid binding of purified and recombinant *Escherichia coli* produced Verocytotoxin *in vitro*. J Biol Chem 1987; **262:** 8834-8839.

173. Head S, Karmali M A, Lingwood C A. Preparation of VT1 and VT2 hybrid toxins from their purified dissociated subunits. Evidence for B subunit modulation of A subunit function. J Biol Chem 1991; **266:** 3617-3621.

174. Igarashi K, Ogasawara T, Ito K, Yutsudo T, Takeda Y. Inhibition of elongation factor I-dependent aminoacyl-tRNA binding to ribosomes by Shiga-like toxin I (VTI) from *Escherichia coli* O157:H7 and by Shiga toxin. FEMS Microbiol Lett 1987; **44:** 91-94.

175. Endo Y, Tsurugi K, Yutsudo T, Takeda Y, Ogasawara T, Igarashi K. Site of action of Verocytotoxin (VT2) from *Escherichia coli* O157:H7 and of Shiga toxin on eukaryotic ribosomes. RNA N-glycosides activity of the toxin. Eur J Biochem 1988; **171:** 45-50.

176. Ogasawara T, Ito K, Igarashi K, Yutsudo T, Nakabayashi N, Takeda Y. Inhibition of protein synthesis by a Verocytotoxin (VT2 or Shiga-like toxin II) produced by *Escherichia coli* O157:H7 at the level of elongation factor 1 -dependent aminoacyl-tRNA building to ribosomes. Microbiol Pathogen 1988; **4:** 127-135.

177. Saxena S K, O'Brien A D, Ackerman E J. Shiga toxin, Shiga-like toxin II variant and ricin are all single-site RNA N-glycosidases of 28S RNA when micro-infected into *Xenopus* oocytes. J Biol Chem 1989; **264:** 596-601.

178. Van de Kar N C A J, Monnens L A H, Karmali M A, van Hinsbergh V W M. Tumour necrosis factor and interleukin-1 induce expression of the Verocytotoxin receptor globotriaosylceramide on human endothelial cells: implications for the pathogenesis of the haemolytic uraemic syndrome. Blood 1992; **80:** 2755-2764.

179. Karmali M A, Steele B T, Petric M, Lim C. Sporadic cases of haemolytic uraemic syndrome associated with faecal cytotoxin and cytotoxin-producing *Escherichia coli* in stools. Lancet 1983; **I(8325):** 619-620.

180. Barrett T J, Green J H, Griffin P M, Pavia A T, Ostroff S M, Wachsmuth I K. Enzyme-linked immunosorbent assays for detecting antibodies to Shiga-like toxin I, Shiga-like toxin II, and *Escherichia coli* O157:H7 lipopolysaccharide in human serum. Curr Microbiol 1991; **23:** 189-195.

181. Maloney M D, Lingwood C A. CD19 has a potential CD77 binding site with a sequence similarity to Verocytotoxin B sub-units: Implications of molecular mimicry for B cell adhesion and enterohaemorrhagic *Escherichia coli* pathogenesis. J Exp Med 1994; **180:** 191-201.

182. Scotland S M, Willshaw G A, Smith H R, Rowe B. Properties of strains of *Escherichia coli* belonging to serogroup O157 with special reference to production of Verocytotoxins VT1 and VT2. Epidemiol Infect 1987; **99:** 613-624.

183. Ostroff S M, Tarr P I, Neill M A, Lewis J H, Hargnett-Bean N, Kobayashi J M. Toxin genotypes and plasmid profiles as determinants of systemic sequelae in *Escherichia coli* O157:H7 infections. J Infect Dis 1989; **160:** 994-999.

184. Tesh V L, Burris J A, Owens J E. Gordon V M, Wadolkowski E A. O'Brien A D, Samuel J E. Comparison of the relative toxicities of shiga-like toxins type I and type II for mice. Infect Immun 1993; **61:** 3392-3402.

185. Gross R J. Verocytotoxin-producing *Escherichia coli* O157. PHLS Microbiol Digest 1990; **7(4):** 119-123.

186. Bitzan M, Richardson S, Huang C, Boyd B, Karmali M A. Patterns and determinants of VT binding to human and animal RBCs *in vitro*. Proceedings of 2nd International Symposium and Workshop on Verocytotoxin (Shiga-like toxin) - producing *Escherichia coli* infections [abstract no. 02.6]; 1994 June; Bergamo, Italy.

187. Kelly J K, Pai C H, Jadusingh I H, Macinnis M L, Shaffer E A, Hershfield N B. The histopathology of rectosigmoid biopsies from adults with bloody diarrhoea due to Verocytotoxin-producing *Escherichia coli*. Amer J Clin Path 1987; **88:** 78-82.

188. Tzipori S, Karch H, Wachsmuth I K, Robins-Browne R M, O'Brien A D, Lior H, *et al*. Role of a 60-megadalton plasmid and Shiga-like toxins in the pathogenesis of infection caused by enterohemorrhagic *Escherichia coli* O157:H7 in gnotobiotic piglets. Infect Immun 1987; **55:** 3117-3125.

189. Dytoc M, Soni R, Cockerill F. de Azavedo J, Louie M, Brunton J, *et al*. Multiple determinants of Verocytotoxin-producing *Escherichia coli* O157:H7: attachment-effacement. Infect Immun 1993; **61:** 3382-3391.

190. Tzipori S, Gibson R, Montanaro J. Nature and distribution of mucosal lesions associated with enteropathogenic and enterohemorrhagic *Escherichia coli* in piglets and the role of plasmid-mediated factors. Infect Immun 1989; **57:** 1142-1150.

191. Hall G A, Dorn C R, Chanter N, Scotland S M, Smith H R, Rowe B. Attaching and effacing lesions *in vivo* and adhesion to tissue culture cells of Verocytotoxin-producing *Escherichia coli* belonging to serogroups O5 and O103. J Gen Microbiol 1990; **136:** 779-786.

192. Pai C H, Kelly J K. Meyers G L. Experimental infection of infant rabbits with Verocytotoxin-producing *Escherichia coli*. Infect Immun 1986; **51:** 16-23.

193. Moon H W, Whipp S C, Argenzio R A, Levine M M, Gianella R A. Attaching and effacing activities of rabbit and human enteropathogenic *Escherichia coli* in pig and rabbit intestines. Infect Immun 1983; **41:** 1340-1351.

194. Donnenberg M S, Kaper J B. Enteropathogenic *Escherichia coli*. Infect Immun 1992; **60:** 3953-3961.

195. Louie M, de Azavedo J C S, Handelsman M Y C, Clark C G, Ally B, Dytoc M, *et al*. Expression and characterisation of the *eae*A gene product of *Escherichia coli* serotype O157:H7. Infect Immun 1993; **61(10):** 4085-4092.

196. Sherman P, Cockerill F, Soni R, Brunton J. Outer membranes are competitive inhibitors of *Escherichia coli* O157:H7 adherence to epithelial cells. Infect Immun 1991; **59:** 890-899.

197. Knutton S, Baldwin T, Williams P H, McNeish A S. Actin accumulation at sites of bacterial adhesion to tissue culture cells: basis of a new diagnostic test for enteropathogenic and enterohaemorrhagic *Escherichia coli*. Infect Immun 1989; **57:** 1290-1298.

198. Bentin L, Montenegro M A, Orskov I, Orskov F, Prada J, Zimmermann S, *et al.* Clone association of Verocytotoxin (Shiga-like toxin) production with enterohaemolysin production in strains of *Escherichia coli*. J Clin Microbiol 1989; **27:** 2559-2564.

199. From the centers for disease control and prevention. Update: multistate outbreak of *Escherichia coli* O157:H7 infections from hamburgers - Western United States, 1992-1993. J Amer Med Assoc 1993; **269(17):** 2194-2196.

200. Samadpour M, Grimm L M, Desai B, Dalia A, Ongerth J E, Tarr P. Molecular epidemiology of *Escherichia coli* O157:H7 strains by bacteriophage restriction fragment length polymorphism analysis: Application to a multistate foodborne outbreak and a day-care centre cluster. J Clin Microbiol 1993; **31:** 3179-3183.

201. Okrend A J G, Rose B E, Matner R. An improved screening method for the detection and isolation of *Escherichia coli* O157:H7 from meat, incorporating the 3M Petrifilm™ TM test kit- HEC-for haemorrhagic *Escherichia coli*. J Food Protect 1990; **53(11):** 936-940.

202. Kim M S, Doyle M P. Dipstick immunoassay to detect enterohaemorrhagic *Escherichia coli* O157:H7 in retail ground beef. Appl Environ Microbiol 1992; **58(5):** 1764-1767.

203. Hollingsworth J. Role of Federal Agencies in controlling *Escherichia coli* O157:H7. Food Safety from farm to table. Pop Med News 1993; **6:** 10-11.

204. United States Department of Agriculture, Food Safety and Inspection Service. Nationwide Beef Microbiological Baseline Data Collection Programme: Steers and Heifers, October 1992 - September 1993, 1994 Jan; 1-39.

205. United States Department of Agriculture, Food Safety and Inspection Service Pathogen Reduction Program: The War on Pathogens, 1993.

206. United States Department of Agriculture, Food Safety and Inspection Service: Mandatory Safe Handling statements on labelling of raw meat and poultry products. (9 CFR Parts 317 and 381). Federal Register 1993 Aug; **58(156):** 43478-43487.

207. USA report: Bacteria warning labels for raw meat and poultry. EC Food Law, 1993 Sept; 23.

208. Centers for Disease Control and Prevention/National Centre for Infectious Disease Division of Bacterial and Mycotic Diseases: "Preventing foodborne illness: *Escherichia coli* O157:H7"; April 1993. [leaflet]

209. de Boer E, van Heerwaarden C, Heuvelink A, Wernars K. Examination of meats for *Escherichia coli* serotype O157:H7. Food Micro '93: 15th International Symposium, The International Committee on Food Microbiology and Hygiene [abstract no.P6-12]; 1993, Aug 31 - Sept 3.

210. Farmer J J, Davis B R. H7 antiserum-sorbitol fermentation medium for detecting *Escherichia coli* O157:H7 associated with haemorrhagic colitis. J Clin Microbiol 1985; **22:** 620-625.

211. Smith H R, Scotland S M. Isolation and identification methods for *Escherichia coli* O157 and other Verocytotoxin-producing strains. J Clin Pathol 1993; **46:** 10-17.

212. Chapman P A, Wright D J, Giddons C A. A comparison of immunomagnetic separation and direct culture for the isolation of Verocytotoxin-producing *Escherichia coli* O157 from bovine faeces. J Med Microbiol 1994; **40(6):** 424-427.

213. Chapman P A. Isolation, identification and typing of Verocytotoxin-producing *Escherichia coli* O157. PHLS Microbiol Digest 1994; **11(1):** 13-17.

214. Chapman P A, Siddons C A, Zadik P M, Jewes L. An improved selective medium for the isolation of *Escherichia coli* O157. J Med Microbiol 1991; **35:** 107-110.

215. Okrend A J G, Rose B E, Lattuada C P. Use of 5-bromo-4-chloro-3-indoxyl-ß-D-glucuronide in MacConkey sorbitol agar to aid in the isolation of *Escherichia coli* O157:H7 from ground beef. J Food Protect 1990; **53:** 941-943.

216. Thompson J S, Hodge D S, Borczyk A A. Rapid biochemical test to identify Verocytotoxin-positive strains of *Escherichia coli* serotype O157. J Clin Microbiol 1990; **28:** 2165-2168.

217. Scotland S M, Cheasty T, Thomas A, Rowe B. Beta-glucuronidase activity of Verocytotoxin-producing strains of *Escherichia coli*, including serogroup O157, isolated in the United Kingdom. Lett Appl Microbiol 1991; **13:** 42-44.

218. Zadik P M, Chapman P A, Siddons C A. Use of tellurite for the selection of Verocytotoxigenic *Escherichia coli* O157. J Med Microbiol 1993; **39:** 155-158.

219. Aleksic S, Karch H, Böckemühl J. A biotyping scheme for Shiga-like (Vero) cytotoxin-producing *Escherichia coli* O157 and a list of serological cross-reactions between O157 and other Gram-negative bacteria. Zbl Bakt 1991; **276:** 221-230.

220. Gunzer F, Böhm H, Rüssmann H, Bitzan M, Aleksic S, Karch H. Molecular detection of sorbitol-fermenting *Escherichia coli* O157 in patients with haemolytic-uraemic syndrome. J Clin Microbiol 1992; **30:** 1807-1810.

221. Okrend A J G, Rose B E, Bennett B. A screening method for the isolation of *Escherichia coli* O157:H7 from ground beef. J Food Protect 1990; **53(3):** 249-52.

222. Szabo R A, Todd E C D, Jean A. Method to isolate *Escherichia coli* O157:H7 from food. J Food Protect 1986; **49:** 768-72.

223. Organon Teknika. EHEC-TEK™. For Detection of *Escherichia coli* O157:H7. Organon Tehnika Corporation, Durham, N. Carolina, 1993 Feb.

224. Okrend A J G, Rose B E, Lattuada C P. Isolation of *Escherichia coli* O157:H7 using O157 specific antibody coated magnetic beads. J Food Protect 1992; **55:** 214-217.

225. Park C H, Hixon D L, Morrison W L, Cook C B. Rapid diagnosis of enterohaemorrhagic *Escherichia coli* O157:H7 directly from faecal specimens using immunofluorescence stain. Amer J Clin Pathol 1994; **101:** 91-94.

226. Lior H, Borczyk A A. False positive identification of *Escherichia coli* O157. Lancet 1987; **I(8528):** 333.

227. Scotland S M, Day N P, Rowe B. Production of cytotoxin affecting Vero cells by strains of *Escherichia coli* belonging to traditional enteropathogenic serogroups. FEMS Microbiol Lett 1980; **7:** 15-17.

228. Smith H R, Willshaw G A, Scotland S M, Thomas A, Rowe B. Properties of Verocytotoxin-producing *Escherichia coli* isolated from human and non-human sources. Zbl Bakt 1993; **278:** 436-444.

229. Karmali M A, Petric M, Lim C, Cheung R, Arbus G S. Sensitive method for detecting low numbers of Verocytotoxin-producing *Escherichia coli* in mixed cultures by use of colony sweeps and polymyxin extraction of Verocytotoxin. J Clin Microbiol 1985; **22:** 614-619.

230. Scotland S M, Rowe B, Smith H R, Willshaw G A, Gross R J. Verocytotoxin-producing strains of *Escherichia coli* from children with haemolytic uraemic syndrome and their detection by specific DNA probes. J Med Microbiol 1988; **25:** 237-243.

231. Basta M, Karmali M, Lingwood C. Sensitive receptor-specified enzyme linked immunosorbent assay for *Escherichia coli* Verocytotoxin. J Clin Microbiol 1989; **27:** 1617-1622.

232. Acheson D W K, Keusch G T, Lightowlers M, Donohue-Rolfe A. Enzyme-linked immunosorbent assay for Shiga toxin and Shiga-like toxin II using P1 glycoprotein from hydatid cysts. J Infect Dis 1990; **161:** 134-137.

233. Downes F P, Green J H, Greene K, Strockbine N A , Wells J G, Wachsmuth I K. Development and evaluation of enzyme-linked immunosorbent assays for detection of Shiga-like toxin I and Shiga-like toxin II. J Clin Microbiol 1989; **27:** 1292-1297.

234. Willshaw G A, Smith H R, Scotland S M, Rowe B. Cloning of genes determining the production of Verocytotoxin by *Escherichia coli*. J Gen Microbiol 1985; **131:** 3047-3053.

235. Willshaw G A, Smith H R, Scotland S M, Field A M, Rowe B. Heterogeneity of *Escherichia coli* 'phages encoding Verocytotoxins: comparison of cloned sequences determining VT1 and VT2 and development of specific gene probes. J Gen Microbiol 1987; **133:** 1309-1317.

236. Thomas A, Smith H R, Willshaw G A, Rowe B. Non-radioactively labelled polynucleotide and oligonucleotide DNA probes for selectively detecting *Escherichia coli* strains producing Verocytotoxin VT1, VT2 and VT2 variant. Mol Cell Probes 1991; **5:** 129-135.

237. Karch H, Meyer T. Single primer pair for amplifying segments of distinct Shiga-like toxin genes by polymerase chain reaction. J Clin Microbiol 1989; **27:** 2751-2757.

238. Scotland S M, Smith H R, Willshaw G A, Rowe B. Verocytotoxin production in strains of *Escherichia coli* is determined by genes carried on bacteriophage. Lancet 1983; **II(8343):** 216.

239. O'Brien A D, Newland J W, Miller S F, Holmes R K, Smith H W, Formal S B. Shiga-like toxin-converting 'phages from *Escherichia coli* strains that cause haemorrhagic colitis or infantile diarrhoea. Science 1984; **226:** 694-696.

240. Scotland S M, Smith H R, Rowe B. Two distinct toxins active on Vero cells from *Escherichia coli* O157. Lancet 1985; **II(8460):** 885-886.

241. Schmitt C K, McKee M L, O'Brien A D. Two copies of Shiga-like toxin II-related genes common in enterohaemorrhagic *Escherichia coli* are responsible for the antigenic heterogeneity of the O157:H- strain E32511. Infect Immun 1991; **59:** 1065-1073.

242. Weinstein D L, Jackson M P, Samuel J E, Holmes R K, O'Brien A D. Cloning and sequencing of a Shiga-like toxin type II variant from an *Escherichia coli* strain responsible for edema disease of swine. J Bacteriol 1988; **170:** 4223-4230.

243. Gross R J, Rowe B. Serotyping of *Escherichia coli*. In: Sussman M, editor. The virulence of *Escherichia coli*. Reviews and Methods. London: Academic Press. 1985; 345-363.

244. Ahmed R, Bopp C, Borczyk A, Kasatiya S. 'Phage-typing scheme for *Escherichia coli* O157:H7. J Infect Dis 1987; **155:** 806-809.

245. Khakhria R, Duck D, Lior H. Extended 'phage-typing scheme for *Escherichia coli* O157:H7. Epidemiol Infect 1990; **105:** 511-520.

246. Frost J A, Cheasty T, Thomas A, Rowe B. 'Phage-typing of Verocytotoxin-producing *Escherichia coli* O157 isolated in the United Kingdom: 1989-91. Epidemiol Infect 1993; **110:** 469-475.

247. Frost J A, Smith H R, Willshaw G A, Scotland S M, Gross R J, Rowe B. 'Phage-typing of Verocytotoxin (VT) producing *Escherichia coli* O157 isolated in the United Kingdom. Epidemiol Infect 1989; **103:** 73-81.

248. Tyler S D, Johnson W M, Lior H, Wang G, Rozee K R. Identification of Verocytotoxin type 2 variant B subunit genes in *Escherichia coli* by the polymerase chain reaction and restriction fragment length polymorphism analysis. J Clin Microbiol 1991; **29:** 1339-1343.

249. Thomas A, Smith H R, Rowe B. Use of digoxigenin-labelled oligonucleotide DNA probes for VT2 and VT2 human variant genes to differentiate Verocytotoxin-producing *Escherichia coli* strains of serogroup O157. J Clin Microbiol 1993; **31:** 1700-1703.

250. Whittam T S, Wolfe M L, Wachsmuth I K, Orskov F, Orskov I, Wilson R A. Clonal relationships among *Escherichia coli* strains that cause haemorrhagic colitis and infantile diarrhoea. Infect Immun 1993; **61:** 1619-1629.

251. Böhm H, Karch H. DNA fingerprinting of *Escherichia coli* O157:H7 strains by pulsed-field gel electrophoresis. J Clin Microbiol 1992; **30:** 2169-2172.

252. Harsono K D, Kaspar C W, Luchansky J B. Comparison and genomic sizing of *Escherichia coli* O157:H7 isolates by pulsed field gel electrophoresis. Appl Environ Microbiol 1993; **59:** 3141-3144.

253. Rietra P J G M, Willshaw G A, Smith H R, Field A M, Scotland S M, Rowe B. Comparison of Verocytotoxin-encoding 'phages from *Escherichia coli* of human and bovine origin. J Gen Microbiol 1989; **135:** 2307-2318.

254. Chart H, Scotland S M, Rowe B. Serum antibodies to *Escherichia coli* O157:H7 in patients with haemolytic uraemic syndrome. J Clin Microbiol 1989; **27:** 285-290.

255. Greatorol J S, Thorne G M. Humoral immune responses to Shiga-like toxin and *Escherichia coli* O157 lipopolysaccharide in haemolytic uraemic syndrome patients and healthy subjects. J Clin Microbiol 1994; **32:** 1172-1178.

256. Chart H. Serodiagnosis of infections caused by *Escherichia coli* O157:H7 and other VTEC. Serodiagn Immunother Infect Dis 1993; **5(1):** 8-12.

257. Chart H, Rowe B. Serological identification of infection by Verocytotoxin-producing *Escherichia coli* in patients with haemolytic uraemic syndrome. Serodiagn Immunother Infect Dis 1990; **4(6):** 413-418.

258. Scotland S M, Said B, Thomas A, Rowe B. Ability of human sera to neutralise the activity of Verocytotoxins VT1, VT2 and variant forms of VT2. FEMS Microbiol Lett 1994; **115:** 285-290.

259. Gunzer F, Karch H. Expression of A and B subunits of Shiga-like toxin II as fusions with glutathione S-transferase and their potential for use in sero epidemiology. J Clin Microbiol 1993; **31:** 2604-2610.

260. Karmali M A, Petric M, Winkler M, Bielaszewska M, Brunton J, van de Kar N, *et al.* Enzyme-linked immunosorbent assay for detection of immunoglobulin G antibodies to *Escherichia coli* Verocytotoxin 1. J Clin Microbiol 1994; **32:** 1457-1463.

261. Council Directive 92/46/EEC, Official J Number L268. 14.09.92.

262. Dairy Products (Hygiene) Regulations. S I No. 1086. London: HMSO 1995.

263. Fresh Meat (Hygiene and Inspection) Regulations. S I No. 539. London: HMSO 1995.

264. Pierard D, Huyghens L, Lauwers S. Diarrhoea associated with *Escherichia coli* producing porcine oedema disease verotoxin. Lancet 1991; **338(8769):** 762

Printed in the United Kingdom for HMSO.
Dd.0298653, 5/95, C15, 3400, 5673, 324746.